D0075477

Larry VandeCreek, DMin
Editor

Spiritual Care for Persons with Dementia: Fundamentals for Pastoral Practice

Spiritual Care for Persons with Dementia: Fundamentals for Pastoral Practice has been co-published simultaneously as *Journal of Health Care Chaplaincy*, Volume 8, Numbers 1/2 1999.

Pre-publication
REVIEWS,
COMMENTARIES,
EVALUATIONS . . .

"**T**he effect of the essays on readers is first evocative: Uncle George, after his stroke, mistaking daughter-in-law Doris for Doloros, his secretary at the bank; Charles holding a tattered photograph of himself beside a P-38 trainer, recounting war stories from 40 years ago, unable to remember where he'd been that morning; a pastor watching from the door to the hospital room as Deacon Chet strokes Agnes' hand, wondering whether Chet has become in her mind her father, or a husband or son she never had.

Then the essays provide fresh air: that the root of our word 'prayer' is Latin 'precari,' which also gave 'precarious' to the language; that chaplains and caregivers need not serve only as reality tests in the here and now, but are permitted, as allowed by persons with dementia, to enter with them into their memories to offer joy or pleasure, forgiveness or support; that deep forgetting, a terrible loss, can offer the compensation of being able to more fully devote oneself to the present, to a maple turning in autumn, or a dogwood coming to filigree in spring.

As promised by Editor Larry VandeCreek, chapters also appeal to the cognition of chaplains and caregivers. Pastors leading worship in care centers are offered a framework for serving persons with dementia, and given insights into the value of visits. Chaplains to staff of long-term care institutions receive a model for assisting staff members to mark deaths and grieve. End notes in each essay are adequate and helpful. Overall, VandeCreek's collection ushers village priests into contemporary scholarship on ministry with persons with ADRD, and encourages continuing research on effective ministry with those persons, who represent not a small or insignificant portion of the body of Christ."

William R. Leety, MA
Pastor
Overbrook Presbyterian Church

"**D**ementia is the story of losses. Losses come in many forms as noted in several articles. Among them are the losses experienced through the process of 'forgetting.' The reasons are many as indicated throughout this volume. Pastoral Care/Caregiving is how we go about re-membering. It is an activity done by family members, caregivers, pastors, and the community. We are all instruments through whom God also re-members. Those of us who still can remember are called to. Just because a person has dementia and forgets, doesn't mean we should. We are called to be present, 'to remember for her/him.'

It is suggested that our responses are to be geared to what is healing rather than what may be harmful. We are to look for points of 'connectedness' and expressions of feelings in the 'now' that can guide us in giving of care. This gives dignity to those who are served by those who minister as God's servants. Dignity is given in our presence, not in our absence. This may call upon us to confront our own fears and limitations. (These articles invite and challenge us to use more than our intellect as the point of effecting relationship and to discover other avenues through which ministry is provided.)

So along with worship opportunities we include 'touch, music, presence, love, smell, color, play, pets, humor, and nature.' As the number of persons with ADRD grow, we too need to grow in developing our abilities to reach out to those whose limits increase as their dementia progresses. The words 'do this in remembrance of me' take on a whole new meaning."

Rev. David H. Pflieger, BCC
Chaplain
The Lutheran Home at Kane, PA

"*Spiritual Care for Persons with Dementia: Fundamentals for Pastoral Practice* is a gold mine of information about the theory and application of pastoral care with persons suffering from dementia. Aimed at chaplains who serve in institutional settings, it is a rich collection of articles and reviews of the literature pertaining to pastoral care and dementia, including the theology that grounds our reason for providing such care.

It will serve as a manual for all who want to address the spiritual needs of cognitively impaired persons who require a special kind of pastoral care that is guided by an understanding of the progression of the disease and the approaches which best communicate the love of God to persons at each stage. Most helpful for me were the chapters in the book which present various demonstrated strategies and suggestions for pastoral care interventions that take advantage of the patient's ability to perform overlearned or habitual tasks, primary motor and sensory functions, emotional awareness, remote memory, and tendency to perseverate. The use of symbols, liturgy, singing, and stories are well-described, as are examples of various worship formats and tools such as reminiscence packets.

While the book deals principally with dementia, it also includes two excellent chapters dealing with protocols and rituals for honesty and gently dealing with the death and remembrance of residents in long-term care facilities."

Rev. David C. Baker, PhD
Director of Chaplaincy Services
LAS Passavant
Retirement Community
Zelienople, PA

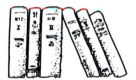

"This 'publication' on providing spiritual care to persons with dementia lives up to its title admirably. The range and scope of the chapters can provide the reader with a basic understanding of everything from the theoretical/theological issues to practical and interactive program suggestions. The overriding themes that become more clear the further one reads in this collection include: (1) the ongoing and undeniable humanness and spiritually full personhood throughout the course of the dementia, (2) the challenge to care providers in recognizing this humanness and spiritual person, and (3) the need to learn to recognize that spiritual connection comes most fully when the world and 'language' of the person with dementia is accepted and understood.

Each of the chapters is rich with insights, illustrative stories and vignettes, and practical guidelines and suggestions."

Rabbi Samuel R. Seicol, MAHL
Director of Religious Services
Hebrew Rehabilitation Center for the Aged
Boston, MA

Spiritual Care
for Persons with Dementia:
Fundamentals
for Pastoral Practice

Spiritual Care for Persons with Dementia: Fundamentals for Pastoral Practice has been co-published simultaneously as *Journal of Health Care Chaplaincy,* Volume 8, Numbers 1/2 1999.

The *Journal of Health Care Chaplaincy* Monographic "Separates"

Below is a list of "separates," which in serials librarianship means a special issue simultaneously published as a special journal issue or double-issue *and* as a "separate" hardbound monograph. (This is a format which we also call a "DocuSerial.")

"Separates" are published because specialized libraries or professionals may wish to purchase a specific thematic issue by itself in a format which can be separately cataloged and shelved, as opposed to purchasing the journal on an on-going basis. Faculty members may also more easily consider a "separate" for classroom adoption.

"Separates" are carefully classified separately with the major book jobbers so that the journal tie-in can be noted on new book order slips to avoid duplicate purchasing.

You may wish to visit Haworth's website at . . .

http://www.haworthpressinc.com

. . . to search our online catalog for complete tables of contents of these separates and related publications.

You may also call 1-800-HAWORTH (outside US/Canada: 607-722-5857), or Fax 1-800-895-0582 (outside US/Canada: 607-771-0012), or e-mail at:

getinfo@haworthpressinc.com

Spiritual Care for Persons with Dementia: Fundamentals for Pastoral Practice, edited by Larry VandeCreek, DMin, BCC (Vol. 8, No. 1/2, 1999). *Offers you a better understanding of dementia and how to better serve persons with this frustrating and often confusing disease.*

Scientific and Pastoral Perspectives on Intercessory Prayer: An Exchange Between Larry Dossey, M.D. and Health Care Chaplains, edited by Larry VandeCreek, DMin (Vol. 7, No. 1/2, 1998). *"Anyone who wonders about our prayers and our needs will be drawn into these dialogues." (Laland E. Elhard, PhD, Professor of Pastoral Theology, Trinity Lutheran Seminary, Columbus, Ohio) Summarizes Larry Dossey's work on prayer and challenges chaplains to think seriously about its role in their ministry.*

Ministry of Hospital Chaplains: Patient Satisfaction, edited by Larry VandeCreek, DMin, and Marjorie A. Lyon (Vol. 6, No. 2, 1997). *Explores patient satisfaction with the general hospital chaplain's ministry.*

Organ Transplantation in Religious, Ethical, and Social Context: No Room for Death, edited by William R. DeLong, MDiv, FCOC (Vol. 5, No. 1/2, 1993). *"I recommend this book to anyone working with transplant recipients or donor families." (Sharon Augustine, RN, MS, Heart and Lung Transplant Service, The Johns Hopkins Hospital, Baltimore)*

Health Care Chaplaincy in Oncology, edited by Laurel Arthur Burton, ThD, and George Handzo, MDiv (Vol. 4, No. 1/2, 1993). *"A valuable collection that speaks of the 'Modern' professional chaplain." (Rev. Elaine Hickman, Manager, Chaplaincy Services, Mercy General Hospital; President, The College of Chaplains, Inc.; Vice President, COMISS (Congress on Ministry in Specialized Settings))*

The Chaplain-Physician Relationship, edited by Larry VandeCreek, DMin, and Laurel Arthur Burton, ThD (Vol. 3, No. 2, 1993). *"Recommended to both chaplains and physicians who are searching for ways to overcome the relational distance between the two professions." (The Journal of Pastoral Care)*

Making Chaplaincy Work: Practical Approaches, edited by Laurel Arthur Burton, ThD (Vol. 1, No. 2, 1988). *"Dr. Burton has done a first-class job of bringing together articulate writers whose content has been informed by their daily practice of ministry within healthcare settings." (David E. Latham, Director of Chaplaincy Services, Community United Methodist Hospital, Henderson, Kentucky)*

Spiritual Care
for Persons with Dementia:
Fundamentals
for Pastoral Practice

Larry VandeCreek, DMin
Editor

Spiritual Care for Persons with Dementia: Fundamentals for Pastoral Practice has been co-published simultaneously as *Journal of Health Care Chaplaincy,* Volume 8, Numbers 1/2 1999.

The Haworth Pastoral Press
An Imprint of
The Haworth Press, Inc.
New York • London • Oxford

Published by

The Haworth Pastoral Press, 10 Alice Street, Binghamton, NY 13904-1580 USA

The Haworth Pastoral Press is an imprint of The Haworth Press, Inc., 10 Alice Street, Binghamton, NY 13904-1580 USA.

Spiritual Care for Persons with Dementia: Fundamentals for Pastoral Practice has been co-published simultaneously as *Journal of Health Care Chaplaincy*™, Volume 8, Numbers 1/2 1999.

Cover design by Thomas J. Mayshock Jr.

Library of Congress Cataloging-in-Publication Data

Spiritual Care for Persons with Dementia: Fundamentals for Pastoral Practice / Larry VandeCreek, editor.
     p. cm.
    "Co-published simultaneously as Journal of health care chaplaincy, volume 8, numbers 1/2 1999."
    Includes bibliographical references and index.
    ISBN 0-7890-0690-1 (alk. paper)
    1. Church work with nursing home patients. 2. Senile dementia–Patients–Religious life. I. VandeCreek, Larry.
BV4435.5.S65 1999
259'.419683–dc21
                                   99-12764
                                         CIP

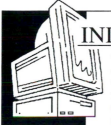

INDEXING & ABSTRACTING

Contributions to this publication are selectively indexed or abstracted in print, electronic, online, or CD-ROM version(s) of the reference tools and information services listed below. This list is current as of the copyright date of this publication. See the end of this section for additional notes.

- *Abstracts in Social Gerontology: Current Literature on Aging*

- *Abstracts of Research in Pastoral Care & Counseling*

- *AgeLine Database*

- *BUBL Information Service: An Internet-based Information Service for the UK higher education community*

- *CNPIEC Reference Guide: Chinese National Directory of Foreign Periodicals*

- *Family Studies Database (online and CD/ROM)*

- *HealthSTAR*

- *Hospital and Health Administration Index*

- *Human Resources Abstracts (HRA)*

- *Leeds Medical Information*

- *Orere Source, The (Pastoral Abstracts)*

- *Religious & Theological Abstracts*

- *Theology Digest (also made available on CD-ROM)*

(continued)

Special Bibliographic Notes related to special journal issues (separates) and indexing/abstracting:

- indexing/abstracting services in this list will also cover material in any "separate" that is co-published simultaneously with Haworth's special thematic journal issue or DocuSerial. Indexing/abstracting usually covers material at the article/chapter level.
- monographic co-editions are intended for either non-subscribers or libraries which intend to purchase a second copy for their circulating collections.
- monographic co-editions are reported to all jobbers/wholesalers/approval plans. The source journal is listed as the "series" to assist the prevention of duplicate purchasing in the same manner utilized for books-in-series.
- to facilitate user/access services all indexing/abstracting services are encouraged to utilize the co-indexing entry note indicated at the bottom of the first page of each article/chapter/contribution.
- this is intended to assist a library user of any reference tool (whether print, electronic, online, or CD-ROM) to locate the monographic version if the library has purchased this version but not a subscription to the source journal.
- individual articles/chapters in any Haworth publication are also available through the Haworth Document Delivery Service (HDDS).

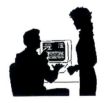

Spiritual Care
for Persons with Dementia:
Fundamentals for Pastoral Practice

CONTENTS

ABOUT THE EDITOR

Larry VandeCreek, DMin, BCC, is Director of Pastoral Research at The HealthCare Chaplaincy in New York City. For the past 23 years, he held faculty and staff positions with The Ohio State University College of Medicine and Public Health and its associated medical center. Dr. VandeCreek is a member of numerous professional associations including the American Association of Marriage and Family Counselors, the Association of Professional Chaplains, Inc., the American Association of Pastoral Counselors, and the Association for Clinical and Pastoral Education. He has published many journal articles which examine aspects of the relationship between religious faith and illness. Dr. Vande-Creek is the author of *A Research Primer for Pastoral Care and Counseling* (Journal of Pastoral Care Publications, 1988) and is Co-Editor of *The Chaplain-Physician Relationship* (1991). He is Editor of the *Journal of Health Care Chaplaincy* (The Haworth Press, Inc.) which has published *Ministry of Hospital Chaplains: Patient Satisfaction* (1997), and *Scientific and Pastoral Perspectives on Intercessory Prayer: An Exchange Between Larry Dossey, M.D. and Health Care Chaplains* (1998).

Preface

Larry VandeCreek, DMin, BCC

If the truth be told, I am afraid of the dementia in my future. Although my family of origin is not particularly plagued with it, I notice my own forgetfulness. "It's probably no worse than 20 years ago," I say to myself reassuringly; "It's just that I'm more anxious about it as I get older." And yet the anxiety does not go away with reassurance.

Dementia is a factor in my wife's family, however, and like most everyone else I will need to cope with it rather directly in the future–either my own or that of someone else. That is one reason for this book; I need to learn more about dementia, how to cope with it, how to minister to those with it, and how to think theologically about it.

This publication is also critically important for other reasons. More people suffer from dementia as the average survival age increases. Are most pastoral caregivers knowledgeable about providing them support and care? Most agree that the answer is "No." Our cognitively oriented culture finds it easy to forget these forgetful persons. Some believe that persons with dementia need little or no pastoral care.

But you may ask, "Are memory and cognitive functions prerequisites for receiving pastoral care?" Of course, they are not prerequisites, but they do pose special challenges. My wife and I have just returned from a visit to relatives which included our attendance at a worship service in a long-term care facility–one of our family members lives there. A guest pastor, himself retired, led the worship on this Pentecost Sunday. The sermon: ten ways in which the Holy Spirit helps us. During the subsequent coffee hour, multiple residents commented that it was

[Haworth indexing entry note]: "Preface." VandeCreek, Larry. Published in *Spiritual Care for Persons with Dementia: Fundamentals for Pastoral Practice* (ed: Larry VandeCreek) The Haworth Pastoral Press, an imprint of The Haworth Press, Inc., 1999, pp. xi-xii. Single or multiple copies of this article are available for a fee from The Haworth Document Delivery Service [1-800-342-9678, 9:00 a.m. - 5:00 p.m. (EST). E-mail address: getinfo@haworthpressinc.com].

impossible to remember all that–nor did I remember it. Surprisingly, they did not seem angry at a pastor who implicitly insulted them by presenting material that relied entirely on memory. It was noted that he literally read the sermon from his manuscript; perhaps that behavior reflected his own memory concerns. Thus it is clear that the usual cognitive methods used in ministry are not helpful (they can, in fact, be hurtful) and new approaches are required. The problem is, as one student recently said, "How can I provide pastoral care when the patient can not carry on a decent conversation?" Reading this book will help answer that question!

The discussion begins with a contribution by Roxanne Miller-Sinclair, a chaplain who describes dementia situations in her clinical setting and theological observations. Jacqueline Stolley, Harold Koenig, and Kathleen Buckwalter then provide more detail about dementia and suggest possible pastoral care approaches. Their contribution is followed by one from Stephen Sapp who presents thorough-going theological considerations, calling us to view persons with dementia "as God sees them." Stephen Post and Peter Whitehouse address additional ethical and pastoral considerations. Three chaplains then make their contributions. David Wentroble and Debbie Everett, both who minister in long-term care facilities, describe their understanding of dementia and pastoral programs which they use. Bethany Knight describes her unique role with nursing homes and the political history of care for the elderly that influences governmental policies. The contribution of Sandra DeForge follows in which she describes memorial services used in the long-term care facility in which she works. I feel less anxious about dementia as I prepare these materials for publication.

We thank all the contributors. May their contributions inform and improve the pastoral care to persons with dementia!

Momma, Oh Momma, I Can't Remember

Roxanne L. Miller-Sinclair, DMin

SUMMARY. Institutionalized persons with dementia present many challenges to pastoral caregivers. The loss of memory and cognitive functions in these persons requires that caregivers value the immediate moment of pastoral contact and ground their ministry in relevant theological foundations. Examples of these challenges are provided and theological concepts are discussed. *[Article copies available for a fee from The Haworth Document Delivery Service: 1-800-342-9678. E-mail address: getinfo@haworthpressinc.com]*

"Momma, Oh Momma," Mr. P. in the Long Term Care unit is crying out loudly. On numerous occasions I have been with him but on this particular day his crying sounds more forlorn than ever before. I have always liked Mr. P. He reminds me of Mr. Magoo in the cartoons; a loving person whose perceptions are amiss but who is likeable nonetheless. But there is one big difference. Mr. Magoo's perception improved when he put on his glasses; Mr. P.'s perception is being steadily eroded by dementia.

I went into the room and asked if I could sit down. "Please, I'm so lonely," he pleaded. I responded, "I know. Your wife will be here in a little while." He asked, "*How* do you know?" I needed to repeat several times throughout the conversation that his wife came every day after lunch.

Roxanne L. Miller-Sinclair is Staff Chaplain, BroMenn Healthcare, Bloomington, IL.

[Haworth co-indexing entry note]: "Momma, Oh Momma, I Can't Remember." Miller-Sinclair, Roxanne L. Co-published simultaneously in *Journal of Health Care Chaplaincy* (The Haworth Pastoral Press, an imprint of The Haworth Press, Inc.) Vol. 8, No. 1/2, 1999, pp. 1-5; and: *Spiritual Care for Persons with Dementia: Fundamentals for Pastoral Practice* (ed: Larry VandeCreek) The Haworth Pastoral Press, an imprint of The Haworth Press, Inc., 1999, pp. 1-5. Single or multiple copies of this article are available for a fee from The Haworth Document Delivery Service [1-800-342-9678, 9:00 a.m. - 5:00 p.m. (EST). E-mail address: getinfo@haworthpressinc.com].

1

"How do you know? I'm so lonely." Then very lucidly he stated, "You gave me the best thing you could . . . your time." Later he said, "My disease is . . . I don't remember things." Then he cried. "Oh, you've given me the best thing," he continued. "God must have sent you. How did you know?" When I reminded him that I visit him often he said, "I don't remember." "I know Mr. P.," I reassured him, "I just wanted to remind you that your wife will be here soon."

As I sat in this holy space with him, I realized how many boundaries had been crossed that day in that room with that person struggling with dementia. I am a Protestant chaplain; he is a faithful Jew. Although he no longer remembers much of his Jewish heritage, God does.

I stopped in again the next day to see him. He smiled brightly, with no memory of my visit the day before. What was important is that God remembers for him. God remembers who we have been as people of faith. I think about God's description of God's self in Scripture, "I Am." For Mr. P. and other persons with dementia, perhaps it is enough to say, "They Are." Even when no other family or friends are living to recall the life of the person with dementia, they continue to be held firmly in God's memory. Within God's memory are all the stories of that person. God, indeed, puts together all an individual's stories so God can see the pattern of the person's life. We have a God who re-members us; a God who takes all the parts and fragments of our life and makes them into a story. God is the ultimate keeper of their memories and we value and care for these persons accordingly.

When Mr. P. cries out "Momma!" it reaches right to the very core of who I am. Such a familiar word—one that a child cries out to his/her mother. When his wife arrives we are never sure if he knows it is his wife or if he thinks it is his momma. Either way, he is comforted by the sight of her face. "Momma!"

This is one example of an interaction with a person with dementia. As with any disease, there are similar patterns and unfamiliar deviations. With Mr. P. as with many others, there are family and friends and members of his faith community who can do his remembering for him. His wife often shares with the staff what he was like prior to his dementia. This is a good way for staff to get glimpses of him.

I am reminded of Ms. A. in another unit who continually talked about her beautiful front porch on her home where she lived as a young girl. Then she would ask for her sister and tell us how angry she was and that her father would kill us. To remind Ms. A. that all of her family died long ago would only traumatize her. It would be for her as if it were the first time she had heard of her family members' deaths. She received peace by telling her visitors about that beautiful front porch because that was reality to her; being a young girl once again at the home place.

I do not enter a person's delusion if I believe it will cause more pain. On one particular occasion, Ms. C. pleaded for someone to telephone her sister. Support staff repeatedly told Ms. C. that her sister had died. Each time they told her was as if she heard it for the first time. Staff persons were trying to be truthful, yet she was traumatized with each telling. Then there was the person whose delusion I would not enter because she was paranoid and thought she was being poisoned by staff.

One individual kept telling me of a recent trip during which she ate so many potatoes. When affirmed, she said she ate sweet potatoes, baked potatoes, and French Fries. For me to tell her she had not been on a recent trip nor had she eaten any potatoes would have been unnecessarily cruel. I believe caregivers need to ask whether the truth will harm or heal in a given situation.

Chaplain Donald K. Nester is a Board Certified Chaplain and an ordained minister in the Mennonite Church. He is a professional colleague with over 25 years of gerontological expertise and states, "I will try to deal with reality until I find that (the patients/residents) are not willing or able to do so, then I will work at entering their delusion."

Another colleague, Chaplain Jim Turner, Jr., also a Board Certified Chaplain and an ordained minister in the Disciples of Christ says, "If there are instances in which I can emotionally connect with the person in reality, I do so. For example, I might say, 'It's a pretty day,' and the person is able to acknowledge that the weather is pleasant. If, however, the person suffering from dementia is talking gibberish and is not in touch with surroundings, then I will try to connect with symbolism." In other words, what is the person trying to say?

As a guide to assessing such situations, caregivers should first make several attempts to discover a person's cognitive and emotional reality on a given day. For example, can the person acknowledge that it is a sunny day? Would the pain of wondering why a loved one has not visited be greater than being reminded graciously and gently that the loved one died some time ago? Both of my colleagues agree with me that one first should assess the situation and then proceed accordingly.

In addition, the unit nurse can describe the person's history as well as previously helpful and harmful interventions. This information is valuable to the chaplain.

Another resident points to my floral print dress and keeps touching the individual flowers and then talks incoherently and points at plants at the nurse's station. Regardless of what her words said or did not say, I thought perhaps she was trying to communicate about gardening. Yet if there was no connection (and I will never know), the fact that that person was noticed and valued was of paramount importance. Why? Because of Jesus' teaching, "Truly I tell you, just as you did it to one of the least of these who are members of my family, you did it to me" (Matthew 25:40, NRSV).

Ministry to those with dementia requires the readiness to be surprised. During each lengthy visit, one gentleman never spoke more than one or two words. However, when a child was brought to visit him during the Christmas season, he looked directly into the child's eyes and asked her if she was excited about Santa Claus. These serendipitous moments are among the most special when ministering with older persons in the long term care setting.

On another unit during December, two residents, both of whom had dementia, were sitting in the hallway conversing with each other about the benefits of leather shoes. Suddenly the conversation changed. One resident turned to the other and asked, "Is it Christmas yet?" The other resident thought for a few moments and replied, "I think it's past." Then, with an air of resignation, the first resident stated, "Damn. I slept through it again!"

Another important area is the education and support of persons with early signs of dementia. During the early diagnosis of dementia, it is important that the individual is given support during their coherent moments so that they can talk about their feelings if they choose. Of equal importance is making available resources for respite for the caregiver(s) such as adult day centers and support groups. At an adult day center, the individual can be left in a safe environment while the caregiver runs errands or works.

Another area of importance in dealing with persons with dementia is continuity. Too much stimulation and too many changes can aggravate and confuse the person. In Jesus' earthly ministry he was consistent with others as he interacted with them.

As we minister with older adults, it is imperative that we develop a theology of aging. In Genesis 1:27, we read that God created woman and man in God's image. If we are created in the image of God, then surely we have some likeness—some bit of the Creator's goodness in us. As children display characteristics handed down from their parents, so all persons have characteristics handed down by the Creator. If all humankind is created in the image of God, then it seems apparent that God's spirit dwells in us throughout the seasons of our lives.

A theory called gerontheology, first coined by Dr. W. Paul Jones (1984), retired professor of philosophical theology at Saint Paul School of Theology in Kansas City, Missouri, is helpful in developing a theology of aging. Jones stressed the notion that gerontology and theology must be considered together. The creation of the term "gerontheology" is his way of emphasizing the need for this interconnectedness.

Henri Nouwen and Walter Gaffney (1974) describe the aging process in terms of a wagon wheel; the cycle of life comes full circle and nearing completion yet continuing to be an integral part of life's process. They state that older persons can be our prophets, showing us the way to our own inevitable aging. They write, "When we have emptied ourselves of false occupations and preoccupations, we can offer free space to old strangers, where not only bread and wine but also the story of life can be shared." This implies that spiritual sustenance is possible through the sharing of the life story.

Indeed, the age-old advice of the Golden Rule equally applies as one deals with persons with dementia. One needs to ask oneself, "How would I like to be treated in the later stages of life if all I had left were memories that didn't make sense to others?" We need to accord value and worth to others simply because they belong to God, knowing that ultimately God holds all our memories.

REFERENCES

Jones, W. Paul. 1984. Gerontheology: Spirituality and aging. *Quarterly papers on religion and aging.* (David B. Oliver, Ed.) Kansas City, MO: Oubri A. Poppele Center for Health and Welfare Studies, Summer, p 3.

Nouwen, Henri, and Walter Gaffney. 1974. *Aging: The fulfillment of life.* Garden City, NY: Image Books, p 14.

Scripture quotations are from the New Revised Standard Version (NRSV).

Pastoral Care for the Person with Dementia

Jacqueline M. Stolley, PhD, RN, CS
Harold Koenig, MD, MHSc
Kathleen C. Buckwalter, PhD, RN, FAAN

SUMMARY. We discuss the various stages of Alzheimer's disease and related disorders (ADRD) and present a psychosocial model which spiritual caregivers can use in their ministry, the Progressively Lowered Stress Threshold (PLST) model. We argue that religious activities are very important to these patients and that spiritual caregivers can make an important contribution. *[Article copies available for a fee from The Haworth Document Delivery Service: 1-800-342-9678. E-mail address: getinfo@ haworthpressinc.com]*

Susan Jones, a 78 year old widow, was admitted to the nursing facility with a diagnosis of dementia of the Alzheimer's type. In the past, Susan, a devout Roman Catholic, worked as a secretary at a Catholic Church in her hometown. She attended daily Mass, prayed

---

Jacqueline M. Stolley is Associate Professor, Trinity College of Nursing, Moline, IL. Harold Koenig is Associate Professor of Psychiatry, Assistant Professor of Internal Medicine, and Director, Center for the Study of Religion/Spirituality and Health, Duke University Medical Center, Durham, NC. Kathleen C. Buckwalter is Professor, College of Nursing and Associate Provost for Health Sciences, University of Iowa, Iowa City, IA.

The names of the patients in this article have been changed to protect their privacy.

[Haworth co-indexing entry note]: "Pastoral Care for the Person with Dementia." Stolley, Jacqueline M., Harold Koenig, and Kathleen C. Buckwalter. Co-published simultaneously in *Journal of Health Care Chaplaincy* (The Haworth Pastoral Press, an imprint of The Haworth Press, Inc.) Vol. 8, No. 1/2, 1999, pp. 7-23; and: *Spiritual Care for Persons with Dementia: Fundamentals for Pastoral Practice* (ed: Larry VandeCreek) The Haworth Pastoral Press, an imprint of The Haworth Press, Inc., 1999, pp. 7-23. Single or multiple copies of this article are available for a fee from The Haworth Document Delivery Service [1-800-342-9678, 9:00 a.m. - 5:00 p.m. (EST). E-mail address: getinfo@haworthpressinc.com].

the Rosary, and regularly participated in Novenas. However she was unable to live alone because of her deteriorating cognition and was placed in a not-for-profit nursing facility with no religious affiliation. This facility is near her son, but 500 miles away from her home community. Susan's religion and beliefs remain very important to her, and are a great source of comfort. However, in her new home, clergy visit only infrequently, and there are no Catholic religious rituals available because of the predominant Scandinavian, Lutheran culture of the rural setting.

Julia Jamieson lives in the same nursing facility, down the hall from Susan. Julia also has dementia, but her dementia is related to multiple small strokes, commonly called multi-infarct or vascular dementia (MID). Because Julia is African-American, she is pre-disposed to having high blood pressure, a condition that contributes to her MID. Julia's Baptist religion is central in her life, and her most frequent visitors are members of her church congregation. These visitors must travel some distance, however, and their visits to Julia occur only monthly. Julia can frequently be heard humming and sometimes singing hymns she remembers from church.

Across the hall resides Rachel Benjamin, who relocated a great distance to this nursing facility to be near her daughter. Rachel is a lifelong member of a Conservative Jewish congregation in a city 150 miles away. Her daughter married outside the faith and no longer practices Judaism, and there are no rabbis in the vicinity of the nursing facility. Like Susan and Julia, Rachel has a diagnosis of dementia, but the type of dementia is not specified.

These three women are unable to safely live alone because of their dementia, and the accompanying cognitive deficits. Even though they come from diverse backgrounds, they have three common concerns: (1) they each have some type of dementia; (2) religion is extremely important in their lives; and (3) their religious needs are not adequately met by clergy because the chaplain who serves the nursing facility is unfamiliar with dementia. However, he is familiar with Susan, Julia and Rachel's various religious orientations, and respects their free expression of religion. The chaplain understands these residents have spiritual needs, even though they are sometimes cognitively and socially inaccessible. Regrettably, care and communication with the person with dementia was not a topic covered in his education for the ministry.

The purpose of this article is to provide an overview of dementia, to present a model of care tailored to these persons and which can be used by any discipline, and to present research that explores the importance of religion and spirituality for persons with dementia. Finally, this article provides questions and hypotheses related to the religious care of persons with dementia which pastoral care specialists can explore and test.

DEMENTIA

Dementia is a chronic disease that affects memory and cognition. Over 70 different disorders can cause dementia, but the Alzheimer's type is the most common, representing 60% to 75% of the elderly who have these problems (Hull, 1996; Jellinger, Danielcyzyk, Fishcher, & Gabriel, 1990). Health care professionals often refer to Alzheimer's disease and related disorders (ADRD), because so many of the dementias have similar manifestations. Therefore, for purposes of this article, dementia will be referred to as ADRD.

Alzheimer's type dementia is a progressive disease and is characterized by memory, intellectual, and language losses, as well as a decline in general competency over a period from 8 to 10 years post diagnosis, ending in death. It is estimated that 10% of individuals between age 65 and 75, and 25% of those over age 85 have the disease (Evans et al., 1989). Other dementias may manifest in a similar manner as Alzheimer's disease, but may also stabilize with adequate treatment. Many persons with dementia are cared for in the home by family members. When family, if available, are no longer able to provide adequate care, the person with dementia is likely placed in a nursing facility. Between 50% and 79% of nursing home residents have some type of dementia; it is a common reason for nursing home placement. Because persons with dementia place many demands on family, institutionalization may be inevitable as the disease progresses.

STAGES OF ADRD

Health care professionals usually describe symptoms of ADRD in stages or phases. For example, Reisberg (1984) described the deterioration of Alzheimer's disease in seven stages, with stage 1 being normal, (no cognitive decline), and stage 7 being late dementia (indicating very severe cognitive decline). Others use a four stage system: forgetfulness, confusion, ambulatory dementia, and the terminal or end stage (Hall & Buckwalter, 1987). It is important to keep in mind that labeling Alzheimer's disease and other dementias in stages can be misleading, because the loss of memory and intellectual abilities is often so gradual that it is difficult to identify when one stage ends and another begins. Also, even though the course of the disease can last more than 10 years, the presentation of memory and cognitive losses varies among ADRD victims, and depends largely upon the extent and location of brain damage. Additionally, the client's pre-morbid personality, support system, and cultural base have an affect on behaviors associated with ADRD (Hall & Buckwalter, 1991).

Forgetful Stage

Loss of short term memory characterizes the "forgetful stage," and the client may use memory aides to compensate. Because he or she is aware that something is wrong with their intellectual functioning, the client can become very depressed, making the forgetfulness seem much worse than it actually is in terms of brain damage. Because the symptoms are not severe, the disease is usually undetectable and not diagnosable at this stage.

Confusion

Memory problems are more evident in the second stage, appropriately labeled "confusion," and the client gradually becomes confused regarding time, place, person, and things. Denial of the memory loss is common, but because of deficiencies in the ability to manage affairs, the cognitive and functional losses become apparent to others. Depression remains a severe risk because the client is afraid of losing his or her mind. To cover for memory loss, the client may make up stories or fabricate responses to questions (confabulate). In addition, problems with memory, judgment, and temper seem more pronounced when the client experiences fatigue. Late in this second stage, the client probably requires assistance in the home, and may need out of home care at an adult day care center to provide respite for family caregivers.

Ambulatory Dementia

As the disease progresses, the client loses the ability to tend to their own personal cares, such as bathing, dressing, and grooming. The ability to reason, communicate verbally, and plan for safety is gradually lost during this third stage of ADRD, called "ambulatory dementia" because the client is often still quite physically robust. Memory loss increases, and although the client may become more withdrawn and self absorbed, the risk for depression lessens, because the client "forgets that he or she forgot." In other words, their impairment is so great that they become less aware of their memory and intellectual problems. With ADRD, the client becomes increasingly unable to cope with stress, and this inability becomes very evident in this third stage. This inability to tolerate stress is manifested in episodes of night wakening, wandering, pacing, increased confusion, belligerence, agitation, withdrawal, and combative behavior. Most nursing facility placement occurs during this stage of ADRD.

Terminal or End Stage

The end stage of the disease occurs as brain damage progresses extensively. In this terminal stage, recognition of family members or even themselves in the mirror is impaired, possibly absent. The loss of the ability to communicate is evident, and the client may become mute or may yell or moan continuously without apparent reason. Purposeful activity levels decline, and the client forgets how to walk. Changes in metabolism, as well as changes in the ability to eat, swallow and chew, may cause the client to lose weight. Because of these changes and impaired mobility, problems related to immobility (e.g., pneumonia, pressure ulcers, and urinary and bowel incontinence) are common. Many persons in this last stage of ADRD develop seizure activity, and most certainly are institutionalized because physical care becomes difficult for family.

PROGRESSIVELY LOWERED STRESS THRESHOLD

Because of memory and intellectual declines, the client with ADRD is unable to accurately perceive and interpret the environment. As a result, behaviors emerge, such as those described above (agitation, combativeness, etc.) (Gerdner, Hall, & Buckwalter, 1996; Hall & Buckwalter, 1987). Repetitive behaviors, such as asking questions over and over, or repeatedly moving an extremity may occur, perhaps because of anxiety or feelings of insecurity. Thus, persons with ADRD require a modified environment because of declining functional and cognitive abilities. The Progressively Lowered Stress Threshold (PLST) model of care, developed by Hall and Buckwalter (1987) contends that persons with ADRD have a declining ability to cope with stress as the disease progresses.

Clients with ADRD exhibit three types of behavior: baseline or normative behavior in which the client is still accessible both cognitively and socially; anxious behavior, which is a reaction to stress; and dysfunctional behavior, when stress is so excessive that the client with dementia cannot process the quantity, complexity, or intensity of stimuli. These behaviors correspond in frequency to the amount of brain damage and the progression of the disease.

Persons with ADRD present with losses in areas other than just memory. These losses are categorized into four symptom clusters: cognitive or intellectual losses, affective or personality losses, conative or planning losses, and progressively lowered stress threshold (Hall & Buckwalter, 1987).

Assumptions and Principles of the PLST Model

Management of the person with ADRD, based on the PLST model, is aimed at providing care that supports the client and compensates for these losses. The PLST model is based on the following assumptions:

- All humans require some control over their person and their environment and need some degree of unconditional positive regard.
- All behavior is rooted and has meaning; therefore, all catastrophic and stress-related behaviors have a cause.
- The confused or agitated client is not comfortable and should be regarded as frightened. All clients have the right to be comfortable.
- The client exists in a 24-hour continuum. Care cannot be planned or evaluated on an 8-hour-shift basis (Hall & Buckwalter, 1987, p. 401; Hall 1991).

Providing measures based on the above assumptions can target symptomatic and supportive activities. Chaplains and pastoral care professionals can use this framework and the following principles to provide effective religious and spiritual care for clients with dementia:

- Maximize the level of safe function by supporting all areas of loss in a prosthetic manner (providing cues to compensate for memory loss)
- Provide the client with unconditional positive regard (accept them as they are, without reservation).
- Use behaviors indicating anxiety and avoidance to determine limits of levels of activity and stimuli.
- Teach others to listen to the client, evaluating verbal and nonverbal responses.
- Modify the environment to support losses and enhance safety.
- Provide ongoing support, care and problem solving for caregivers (Gerdner et al., 1996, p. 243; Hall & Buckwalter, 1987, p. 401; McCloskey & Bulechek, 1996, pp. 201-202).

In the case of Susan, Julia and Rachel, chaplains and pastoral care professionals can reach individuals in various stages of dementing illnesses, preserving their dignity and individuality as well as respecting their religiosity.

The PLST model offers health care a framework for managing persons with ADRD. Six factors seem to cause excess disability or catastrophic behaviors (e.g., withdrawal, agitation, aggression, etc.) for persons with diminishing cognitive functioning. These are fatigue; changes in caregiver, routine or environment; multiple competing stimuli, such as noise, art work, and caffeinated beverages; unrealistic expectations of others; the client's affective response to cognitive loss; and physical stressors such as pain, infection and adverse medication reactions. After discussing research results regarding the importance of religion for persons with dementia, this article will illustrate how pastoral care personnel can incorporate the tenets of the PLST model and dementia management to provide effective religious interventions.

RELIGION, AGING AND DEMENTIA

Research results support the importance of religious activity to older persons in terms of their general physical and mental well-being. Cox and Hammonds (1988) report that although persons in all age groups express a belief in God, the older one grows the more inclined s/he is to express a belief in God. Elders also have a greater proclivity to report that religion is significant in their lives and to believe that there is life after death. Nearly all of the studies that have examined religiosity and life satisfaction came to a similar conclusion–persons with an active religious life report greater life satisfaction and are better adjusted than those who do not. One interpretation of these positive associations is that the church evolves into a focal point of social coherence and activity for the elderly, supplying them with a feeling of community and well-being (Cox & Hammonds, 1988).

Other studies show the importance of religion among different cultural groups. A national sample of 581 older African-Americans revealed that frequency of church attendance was the most important predictor of both frequency and amount of social support (Taylor & Chatters, 1986). Likewise, Krause and Van Tran (1989) studied a nationwide sample of older African-Americans (N = 511) to determine whether religious involvement helped to reduce the negative impact of stressful life events. Their findings indicate that although life stress tends to erode feelings of self-worth and mastery, these negative effects are offset or counterbalanced by increased religious involvement. Walls and Zarit (1991) explored the type of support African-American churches and families provide, and how that support relates to the well-being of the elderly. Findings indicate that the family network is perceived as more supportive than the church network, but that church support contributes to feelings of well-being. Perceptions of support from the churches and not the spiritual aspects of religion or involvement in organized religious activities are associated with well-being (Walls & Zarit, 1991).

RELIGION AND DEMENTIA

Few empirical studies have investigated the relationship between the use of religious beliefs or activities and well-being of persons with cognitive impairments. A study conducted by Koenig and associates (Koenig et al., 1992) documented an inverse relationship between cognitive impairment and religious coping, particularly among those men retired from unskilled labor. This means that religious coping ability diminished with increasing cognitive impairment. This association was recently replicated in a separate study (Koenig et al., 1998).

Reasons for this relationship may be that religion protects persons against developing cognitive declines in later life, or perhaps the impairment of cognitive functioning prohibits the person from using previously learned religious coping skills (Koenig, 1994). While the former explanation cannot be confirmed at this time, the latter explanation is plausible, considering that the ability to read religious literature, pray, listen to sermons and process religious cognitions decline with the loss of cognitive ability. This does not mean, however, that persons with dementia do not receive comfort from participation in religious events. A thorough analysis of the stage of the dementing illness and personal religious history can assist caregivers in planning religious activities that provide comfort and solace even for the most impaired person with dementia and their family members.

While it is usually accepted that religion grows in importance for older people in general, perhaps as a solace for increased isolation and dependency, or as their eventual demise is anticipated, religious activities may be equally important to those with dementia. Even among the frail elderly and the demented there seems to be awareness of a Higher Being and a desire to establish contact (Abramowitz, 1993). In the Melabev clubs for the mentally impaired elderly in Israel, the ritual of prayer in the daily program had therapeutic value. The familiar prayers were comfortable, the activity was respectful, non-threatening, structured and adult-like. They allowed each member to take part at his/her functional level and for certain participants to affirm themselves. The prayers were also a source of stimulation for many and provided an opportunity to enhance a spiritual life (Abramowitz, 1993). Anecdotal reports relayed to the authors suggested that religious activities such as prayer, ritual and music can provide comfort to persons with a dementing illness. While these activities are only a partial expression of religion and religiosity, these findings are important, especially when considering the cognitively impaired elder.

Caregivers of persons with dementia often cite religion and religiosity as helping them cope with the trials of caregiving. Investigators have reported that religious belief was a significant predictor of adaptation to the caregiving experience (Rabins et al., 1990) and that God was a very personal part of the caregiver's support system. To lend credence to these findings, a study conducted in Iowa examining the needs, resources and responses of rural caregivers of persons with Alzheimer's disease reported that rural white caregivers (N = 72) frequently used prayer as a coping mechanism and were motivated by a Christian ethic (Iowa Governor's Report, 1989). The majority of these caregivers (92%) stated that God helped them in their caregiving efforts. While religion was not the primary focus of this study, results confirmed that belief in God and a code of ethics plays an important supportive part in the caregiving role.

Further, other investigations analyzing statements by caregivers revealed that religiosity was a pervasive theme (Whitlatch, Meddaugh, Langhout, 1992). Statements of 31 caregivers were categorized into topic areas based on program objectives and content identified as important to caregiver support, including knowledge of ADRD, caregiving problems and strategies, resources, and feelings. The investigators described religiosity as a possible coping resource expressed by support group members while sharing their family caregiving experiences. Statements were discussed in terms of the Springfield Religiosity Schedule (SRS) (Koenig et al., 1988), categorizing them as either organized religious activity, non-organized religious activity, or intrinsic religiosity. Subjects identified the importance of all three areas of religiosity. The prominence of religion-related discussion among caregivers in this evaluation indicates the need for further research regarding the extent and nature of religiosity as a coping mechanism among caregivers, as well as the investigation of programs that support caregiver access to and participation in religious activity (Whitlatch et al., 1992). It is not surprising, then, that Kaye and Robinson (1994) found that caregiving wives of persons with dementia used spiritual behaviors such as prayer and forgiveness as coping mechanisms more frequently than non-caregiving wives. It follows that if religiosity assists persons with psychological coping, it would play a large role in coping in the caregiving situation.

Stolley (1997) found that caregivers not only identified prayer as an effective coping mechanism, but reported that personal religious activities performed with the care recipient, such as Bible reading and prayer, provided a method of communication that transcended the difficult caregiving process and contributed to effective coping. Furthermore, many of the caregivers in her study identified personal religious activities as strategies they used to cope with the caregiving situation. These included activities that the caregiver performed alone as well as those performed with the care recipient. Thus, in some cases, simple religious activities seemed to provide a sense of comfort to both individuals.

DEMENTIA MANAGEMENT

The PLST model informs the management of persons with dementia. The manner of communication is of primary importance. Language must be simple and straightforward. Exchanges must be very concrete because abstract reasoning is lost. The loss of memory requires that the use of vague pronouns be avoided. For example, when talking to Mrs. Jamieson about her daughter, always refer to her daughter by name, rather than as "she" or "her." Mrs. Jamieson does not have the ability to remember that "she" or "her" refers to her daughter. Other communication strategies include always identifying oneself and the client by name, using good eye contact, and accompanying verbal exchanges with consistent non-verbal language.

The six stress-related causes of excess disability identified earlier can be incorporated into the religious aspect of care.

Fatigue

The person with ADRD may not be in touch with their own level of fatigue. They may continue to be active well beyond the point of exhaustion because they simply do not have the intellectual ability to recognize fatigue. Thus, frequent short (20 to 90 minute) structured rest periods are planned to prevent the person with ADRD from becoming over tired. Additionally, activities and interactions can be planned at a time of day when the client is rested and fresh. Thus, visits by the pastoral care professional can take place at a time when the cognitively impaired client is likely to benefit from them. Although many persons are most rested in the morning, this can differ with individuals, and information related to the person's "best time of day" should be obtained from the caregiver.

Research results show that music can be very therapeutic for persons with dementia, particularly music with which they are familiar and that they enjoy. Thus, a religious activity to incorporate into rest periods could include favorite religious or spiritual music. For Mrs. Jones, a Gregorian Chant may be restful, or perhaps a recording of a Latin Mass. Remember, long term memory remains intact for persons with cognitive impairment until the later stages of dementia and thus Mrs. Jones may remember the pre Vatican II Latin Masses and find comfort in them. Mrs. Jamieson may enjoy spirituals or gospel songs sung in her church. Perhaps her church choir could make a recording of religious songs. For Mrs. Benjamin, recordings of a cantor singing may be soothing and facilitate rest and peace. For each woman, the music intervention may be similar, but different depending on their likes, dislikes, and religious preferences.

Change in Caregiver, Environment or Routine

Because of memory and other intellectual losses, persons with dementia cannot readily store and retrieve new information and it is difficult for a person with dementia to tolerate change. Caregivers must act "prosthetically," that is, provide what has been lost or damaged, by offering security and structure. Many nursing facilities do not rotate staff because it is upsetting for the person with ADRD, and familiar caregivers are a comfort to the person with dementia. Pastoral care professionals can also maximize the structure of religious activities. This can be done by having the same chaplain conduct religious activities with familiar rituals and items. Mrs. Jones may appreciate holy water, a rosary, or a crucifix, Mrs. Jamieson may treasure a simple cross, and Mrs. Benjamin a Star of David or the Jewish Scriptures. Whatever the symbols, they must be congruent with the religious beliefs of the individual and provide comfort and solace.

It may not be possible for the same chaplain to make all visits to the person with dementia. However, it is possible for chaplains to plan visits so that they are predictable and occur at the same time and the same day each week. Although content of visits can vary, it is important to maintain consistency. The structure and rituals provide a sense of security for the person with ADRD, who, because of memory losses, experiences new things from minute to minute. It may also be helpful if the chaplain or pastoral care professional wears traditional religious clothing, such as a Roman collar, so that they are easily recognizable. As noted above, chaplains should identify the client by name and introduce themselves at each visit.

Multiple Competing Stimuli

Because persons with ADRD have difficulty interpreting the environment, stimuli must be kept to a minimum. This does not mean that surroundings should be sterile, but that stimuli should be modified so that the ADRD persons do not have to process several competing activities at once. This includes communication. A simple, short prayer will likely be more comforting than a long religious service that is attended by many people. In fact, persons with ADRD cannot tolerate attendance at a large church that provides many distractions and people. Small gatherings in a small room are probably most beneficial, and activities should be brief, simple, and comforting. Touch can be incorporated into these activities if it is comfortable for the client and the pastoral care professional. It can maximize simple interactions and serve to help the client feel safe, conveying an unconditional positive regard which is a basic assumption of the PLST model.

If participation in a high stimulation activity is desired, it is important to alternate a more low-key activity. For example, if Mrs. Jamieson attends Sunday service at her local church, it may be exhausting and confusing for her to also attend a church pot luck or even go out to a noisy restaurant after services. She would be better served to have a 40 to 90 minute period of rest before becoming involved in another high stimulus activity.

Religious holidays are important to persons of all faiths, and decorations or pictures can help the person with ADRD understand the significant season or religious festival. Holiday decorations, however, should be kept simple and non-toxic. Persons with ADRD frequently consume non-edible items because they do not remember the purpose of the item. Modifying the environment is central to humane care for the person with ADRD.

Unrealistic Expectations and Affective Response to Loss

As the dementia progresses, higher cognitive functioning decreases, and the person with ADRD loses the ability to function in many areas. A grandmother may be unable to tie her shoes, or a former math teacher may lose the ability to do simple addition and subtraction. These losses are very apparent to persons who deal with ADRD clients but are also apparent to the victims themselves particularly in the earlier stages of the disease. The person grieves the loss of their ability to perform even simple tasks, and can become even more depressed when reminded of their losses. Thus, ADRD persons have good and bad days, and their ability to function is affected by these natural fluctuations.

Keeping this in mind, pastoral care professionals can incorporate simple religious activities and guide the person with ADRD in such a way that their dignity and self worth remain intact. As stated previously, for the person with ADRD, simple prayers may be all he or she can manage. The chaplain can say the prayers with the client, not pointing out errors or mispronunciations. Prayers and rituals should be simple and familiar–and comforting.

Because short term memory is impaired and long term memory remains more intact for persons with ADRD, they may refer to times in their past life as if they were current. For example, a 90 year old woman may call out to "Mama," when the institutional staff know that her mother could not possibly be alive. Or, the husband with ADRD may tell his wife he wants to go home when he is in the home he has shared with his wife for 50 years. It is our tendency to orient persons to reality, telling them "Your Mama is dead" or "This is your home." As a result, the person with ADRD may become even more agitated and upset. Rather than orient the person to reality, it is probably better to support their reality and validate their experiences, focusing on the emotional overtones. When the 90 year old asks for "Mama," perhaps providing her with a hug may give her what she needs–the unconditional love and affection of a mother. Rather than telling the husband that "this is your home," talk about his childhood home, and perhaps mention that it is too late to leave, but the matter can be discussed tomorrow. Short term memory loss is merciful in these cases, because by the next morning the person with ADRD has likely forgotten about Mama or going home.

Chaplains and pastoral care professionals may be mistaken for a religious person that the client with ADRD knew in the past. It is important to identify yourself and the client by name with each encounter, but it is not necessary to correct the client with ADRD if they do not recall names and status accurately. Even after being introduced, the person with ADRD may call the chaplain by the name of a beloved pastor from his or her past. Rather than constantly correcting the person and confronting them with their memory losses, it is better to validate their experience and "go with the flow." A religious or spiritual interaction is more positive if there are few reminders of losses, and may be extremely beneficial if the person with ADRD perceives a beloved clergy in a stranger.

Physical Stressors

Persons with ADRD may not be able to interpret simple bodily signals, such as hunger or the need to urinate. Instead, they may become restless and agitated, unable to communicate or relieve their discomfort. Knowing the client with dementia is prone to this, chaplains and pastoral care professionals can call on caregivers to intervene if they suspect that a physical stressor, such as pain, is causing agitation. With relief of the stressor, the encounter can be more effective and rewarding.

Support for Caregivers

Family members frequently care for persons with ADRD until very late in the disease, and family continue to be involved with care after the client with ADRD is admitted to a nursing facility. Chaplains and pastoral care personnel cannot neglect this important relationship, and the impact of a dementing illness on the family. As discussed earlier, caregivers report that they use religious coping strategies and that they are very effective. Pastoral care professionals can include family members in religious activities and provide solace and counseling for them. Other members of the congregation can provide enormous support for family, and the power of private religious activities cannot be overestimated. Very frequently the family is overlooked as an asset in providing care, or even as needing care and support themselves. Family caregivers have noted the importance of religious activities and the perceived lack of formal religious support (Burgener, 1994). Chaplains can take the leading role in including family in religious activities.

CONCLUSION

Chaplains and pastoral care professionals can have a tremendous impact on persons with ADRD and their loved ones. Armed with information gained from the PLST model of dementia care, chaplains can incorporate religious activities to be of greatest benefit to the demented client. For Susan, Julia and Rachel, religious activities can be tailored to fit their religious preference and their level of cognitive functioning. Their religious lives can continue, promoting a continued sense of satisfaction and solace.

Research is ongoing regarding the care and treatment of persons with dementia. Chaplains and pastoral care personnel can participate in these investigations that explore the use of religious music, rituals and other activities in providing comfort (compared with other activities), patterns of religious activities that are most effective, and methods of providing pastoral care to family members and caregivers. With the recent emphasis on religion and spirituality in healing and health care, now is a prime time to establish a research agenda.

REFERENCES

Abramowitz, L. 1993. Prayer as therapy among the frail Jewish elderly. *Journal of Gerontological Social Work*, *19*(3/4), 69-74.

Burgener, S.C. 1994. Caregiver religiosity and well-being in dealing with Alzheimer's dementia. *Journal of Religion and Health*, *33*, 175-189.

Cox, H., & Hammonds, A. 1988. Religiosity, aging, and life satisfaction. *Journal of Religion and Aging*, *5*(1/2), 1-21.

Evans, D.A., Funkenstein, H.H., Albert, M.S., Scherr, P.A., Cook, N.R., Chown, M.J., Hebert, L.E., Hennekens, C.H., & Taylor, J.O. 1989. Prevalence of Alzheimer's disease in a community population of older persons. Higher than previously reported. *JAMA 262*(18), 2551-6.

Gerdner, L. A., Hall, G.R., & Buckwalter, K.C. 1996. Caregiver training. *Image*, *28*(3), 241-246.

Hall, G.R. 1991. Altered though processes: SDAT. In: M. Maas and K. Buckwalter (eds.), *Nursing Diagnoses and Interventions of the Elderly*. Menlo Park, Calif.: Addison-Wesley.

Hall, G.R., & Buckwalter, K.C. 1987. Progressively lowered stress threshold: A conceptual model for care of adults with Alzheimer's disease. *Archives of Psychiatric Nursing*, *1*(6), 309-406.

Hall, G.R., & Buckwalter, K.C. 1991. Clinical outlook: Whole disease care planning. Fitting the program to the client with Alzheimer's disease. *Journal of Gerontological Nursing*, *17*(3), 38-41.

Hull, M. 1996. Oral Presentation, Alzheimer's Conference. Friday Center at Duke University. Chapel Hill, North Carolina.

Iowa Governor's Task Force on Alzheimer's Disease and Related Disorders Final Report. 1989. Des Moines, Iowa.

Jellinger, K., Danielczyk, W., Fischer, P., & Gabriel, E. 1990. Clinicopathological analysis of dementia disorders in the elderly. *Journal of Neurological Science*, *95*, 239-258.

Kaye, J., & Robinson, K.M. 1994. Spirituality among caregivers. *Image: Journal of Nursing Scholarship*, *26*(3), 218-221.

Koenig, H.G., Smiley, M., & Gonzales, J.P. 1988. *Religion, Health, and Aging: A Review and Theoretical Integration*. New York: Greenwood Press.

Koenig, H.G., Cohen, H.J., Blazer, D.G., Pieper, C., Meador, K.G., Shelp, F., Goli,

V., & DiPasquale, R. 1992. Religious coping and depression in elderly hospitalized medically ill men. *American Journal of Psychiatry, 149,* 1693-1700.

Koenig, H.G. 1994. *Aging and God: Spiritual Paths to Mental Health in Midlife and
Later Years.* NY: The Haworth Press, Inc.

Koenig, H.G., Weiner, D.K., Peterson, B.L., Meador, K.G., & Keefe, F.J. 1998.
Religious coping in institutionalized elderly patients. *Internal Journal of Psychiatry in Medicine,* in press.

Krause, N., & Van Tran, T. 1989. Stress and religious involvement among older
blacks. *Journal of Gerontology, 44*(1), S4-13.

McCloskey, J.C., & Bulechek, G.M. 1996. *Nursing Interventions Classification
(NIC),* 2nd Edition. Dementia Management (Intervention #6460, pp. 201ff). St.
Louis: Mosby.

Rabins, P.V., Fitting, M.D., Eastham, J., & Zabora, J. 1990. Emotional adaptation
over time in caregivers for chronically ill elderly people. *Age and Ageing, 19,*
185-190.

Reisberg, B., Ferris, S.H., Arnand, R., DeLeon, M.J., Schneck, M.K., Buttinger, C.,
& Borenstein, J. 1984. Functional staging of dementia of the Alzheimer's type.
Annals of the New York Academy of Science, 435, 481ff.

Stolley, J.M. 1997. Religiosity and coping for caregivers of persons with Alzheimer's
disease and related dementia. Unpublished doctoral dissertation. Iowa City: University of Iowa.

Taylor, R.J., & Chatters, L.M. 1986. Church-based informal support among elderly
blacks. *The Gerontologist, 26*(6), 637-42.

Walls, C.T., & Zarit, S.H. 1991. Informal support from black churches and the
well-being of elderly blacks. *The Gerontologist, 31*(4), 490-495.

Whitlatch, A.M., Meddaugh, D.I., & Langhout, K.J. 1992. Religiosity among Alzheimer's disease caregivers. *The American Journal of Alzheimer's Disease and
Related Disorders & Research,* 7(6), 11-20.

"To See Things as God Sees Them": Theological Reflections on Pastoral Care to Persons with Dementia

Stephen Sapp, PhD

SUMMARY. Although theology is often seen as impractical speculation on unimportant matters, it serves as a necessary foundation–and
provides valuable guidance–for chaplains who must provide pastoral
care to persons with dementia and their families. Theology can help us
"to see things as God sees them." Among the theological doctrines
found in the Hebrew-Christian scriptures and traditions that are particularly helpful are the following: human creation "in the image of God";
human nature as a psychophysical unity; the dependence of all persons
upon God's mercy; the centrality of community; and God's judgment of
personal worth by standards very different from those of "the world."
A model for applying these concepts and some thoughts of the importance of chaplains are offered. *[Article copies available for a fee from The
Haworth Document Delivery Service: 1-800-342-9678. E-mail address: getinfo@
haworthpressinc.com]*

WHY THEOLOGY?

Why does a journal for health care chaplains include an article on
theological reflections in a book on pastoral care and dementia? Chap-

Stephen Sapp is Professor and Chair, Department of Religious Studies, University of Miami, Coral Gables, FL.

[Haworth co-indexing entry note]: "'To See Things as God Sees Them': Theological Reflections on
Pastoral Care to Persons with Dementia." Sapp, Stephen. Co-published simultaneously in *Journal of
Health Care Chaplaincy* (The Haworth Pastoral Press, an imprint of The Haworth Press, Inc.) Vol. 8, No.
1/2, 1999, pp. 25-43; and: *Spiritual Care for Persons with Dementia: Fundamentals for Pastoral Practice*
(ed: Larry VandeCreek) The Haworth Pastoral Press, an imprint of The Haworth Press, Inc., 1999,
pp. 25-43. Single or multiple copies of this article are available for a fee from The Haworth Document Delivery
Service [1-800-342-9678, 9:00 a.m. - 5:00 p.m. (EST). E-mail address: getinfo@haworthpressinc.com].

laincy after all is an intensely practical and results-oriented profession, with precious little time for leisurely reflection. And everyone knows that theology is not first and foremost about acquiring skills that can be immediately applied to tasks or problems as techniques for their accomplishment or solution. Theology, instead, is a way of perceiving the world and the place of human beings in it, of understanding human existence and experience in the context of a set of historical symbols that a particular group of people have come to see as explaining the world better for them than any other ways. Furthermore, it must be granted that theology is popularly seen (insofar as anybody bothers to think about it all!) as some type of abstract, virtually incomprehensible, and certainly not particularly useful speculation undertaken by pointy-headed academics safely ensconced in seminary and university ivory towers.

But to hold such a view of theology (despite some validity to it) is to do the "queen of the sciences" an injustice, even in this scientific, materialistic age. Krister Stendahl, former dean of the Harvard Divinity School, offered a helpful alternative to the popular view of theology when he once said that "to do theology is to try to see things as God sees them." He immediately, appropriately, and necessarily added, "That task is so obviously arrogant and oversized that we can only do it playfully—as children. But to children, play is serious and creative, and it does something to their growth."

One is hesitant in an article dealing with dementia to suggest doing *any*thing "playfully" (though family caregivers are the first to insist that maintaining a sense of humor is essential to coping with such illnesses). Nonetheless, in addition to affirming Stendahl's wise reminder that play can be both creative and essential for healthy maturation, I would argue that the first part of his statement is surely apropos here for the simple reason that all those who call themselves *chaplains* have a clear responsibility to see—not only *things*—but especially their patients/clients as God sees them. And what is true of chaplaincy in general is likely more true of *health care* chaplaincy in particular. In situations of illness and death, human beings are most vulnerable, and even those who do not normally engage in religious reflection or activity often turn to it for strength and solace. So it appears that theology *can* play an important role in chaplaincy.

Indeed, in today's health care system, the physical needs of patients are obviously recognized; that after all is why they are in the system. If the right personnel are available and time permits, patients' psycho-social needs can also be addressed. But all too often their spiritual needs are not recognized or considered legitimate targets for intervention; certainly these needs are not frequently acknowledged and dealt with by medical professionals. Chaplains are therefore critical in the caregiving scheme if *whole* persons are to be the subject of care. And with dementia as with any other illness, spiritual needs–of both the person with dementia and the family caregivers–are very real.

Before looking specifically at what theology might have to offer to those who provide pastoral care to persons with dementia, it is helpful to consider a preliminary issue. If we are to try to "see things as God sees them," it is wise to recall the observation of the old hillbilly that "what you see depends on where you stand," an idea expressed many centuries earlier by that great Jewish compendium of wisdom, the Talmud, in slightly different words: "We do not see things as *they* are; we see them as *we* are." The way we treat persons with dementia is obviously determined by what we think of them–how we see them –and that in turn depends to a very large degree upon how we see *ourselves*. Indeed, I will probably spend at least as much time in this article addressing this issue as I will looking at those with dementia. I have suggested that one practical contribution theology has to make to pastoral care is encouragement to see things, and particularly other people, as God sees them; I will keep constantly before us also the admonition to strive to be aware of where we stand as we do that. In short, it is my firm conviction that the most important thing professionals bring to the work place is their values because these values drive what professionals do and how they do it. I must note at this point that I stand in the Reformed Christian tradition and therefore see the world from that particular faith perspective. I believe, however, that what I say in this article has application to other traditions as well. The language, examples, and perhaps even justifications will differ, but the fundamental points are affirmed in one way or another by virtually all the major faith traditions I know.

A related point is important in this regard, going a little beyond dementia care alone, and this has to do with another aspect of how we see ourselves. A great deal of research is becoming available about the link between religion (or spirituality) and health, providing "scientif-ic" evidence that supports the crucial nature of the role of chaplains. Again, what is true of health in general is perhaps even more true of aging and the maladies associated with it (at least insofar as *every*one will age and thus be forced to confront his or her mortality, whereas not everyone will face serious illness earlier in life).[1] Thus those who approach aging and the issues it raises including the problems present-ed by Alzheimer's disease (AD)–from a religious point of view–have absolutely no reason to feel inferior or apologetic, even if the broader disciplines of geriatrics and gerontology within which they work (not to mention managed care administrators) may look askance at them and sometimes even question their ministry or the need for it.

In fact, chaplains offer something that scientific medicine cannot provide but that is desperately needed today. We have to remember constantly that the meaning of old age, of disease in general, and certainly of AD is inevitably linked to the meaning of life itself, and that is simply not a scientific question. It is the radically *theological* question about the very nature and purpose of human life. Science may be able to provide us the *means* to live longer and healthier lives, but it is utterly powerless to offer us any *meaning* to live for. The question that contemporary scientific gerontology faces–certainly on the practical level–is therefore precisely the question to which religious faith claims to have the answer. So it is worth remembering that science and the gerontological specialties built upon it–for all their wonderful contributions–simply cannot provide what we really need as we age and especially as we face such a terrible assault on our identity and understanding of good and evil as AD, namely, the mean-ing of it all. But religion can offer precisely that, and those who represent religious traditions must offer it.

One final word on this matter, with both a general and a particular application: University of Chicago theologian David Tracy has aptly reminded us that human existence is marked by three inescapable characteristics: finitude (we will age and die); contingency (accidents happen); and transience (everything changes). In a general sense, un-less we acknowledge this reality and are able to accept our *own* mortality, we cannot possibly accompany *others* on their journey of aging because for them it necessarily leads to death. If we cannot face that fact for ourselves we will simply not be able really to be there with them as they have no choice but to face it. And what is true in general is equally true in the particular case of dementia: It is admittedly very difficult to be faithful in providing pastoral care to one who is sinking into cognitive quicksand when virtually all the tools available in one's tool kit depend on the ability to function cognitively and to relate on that level. But however one comes to see persons with dementia, it remains inescapably true that to provide meaningful pastoral care to persons with dementia demands that the chaplain be creative and extend his or her repertoire of helping techniques beyond those based on rational conversation and the ability to remember.

Dementia, of course, is all about memory, or actually the loss of it (at least in the popular understanding–"Oh, no! I've lost my car keys again. I must have Alzheimer's!"). Thus dementia raises questions for "memory-based" religions like Judaism, Christianity, and Islam that are even more difficult to deal with than those presented by other diseases, as troublesome as they may be. If remembering is essential for one to practice a religion, what happens when a person can no longer remember–not the meaning of the *seder* or of the doctrine of justification by grace alone–but even his or her own name? Is such a person no longer of worth to such a religion? No longer of value to a God who–one could argue–in a very real sense *exists* precisely *in the memory* of that God's followers? Now we turn to the theological traditions of Judaism and primarily Christianity to see what guidance we can find there in the face of such questions.

SOME BASIC THEOLOGICAL CONCEPTS

Several concepts[2] from the Hebrew-Christian scriptures seem to me especially appropriate in helping us to "see things as God sees them" with regard to pastoral care of persons with dementia (after all, depending on one's view of the inspiration of scripture, it can be argued that these writings express the way God *does* see things!). I do not have the space to develop a complete biblical hermeneutic here or to explicate each doctrine fully. Also, as I said earlier, though I believe each concept can find some degree of common acceptance among those from different traditions, I am well aware that interpretations of these doctrines will vary. Nonetheless, these ideas can serve as a basic foundation from which we may begin to try to see both ourselves and others as God sees us and them.

CREATION "IN THE IMAGE OF GOD"

The first theological concept of help to us in this context is an idea that appears in the very first chapter of the scriptures common to

Judaism and Christianity, namely, the creation of human beings *imago Dei,* in God's own image, according to God's likeness (Genesis 1:26-27). Given the prohibition in Hebrew religion of "graven images" (Exodus 20:4)–perhaps growing out of the desire to emphasize that this God was not a local deity with physical form but a cosmic being not so limited–finding this language in such a critical passage is somewhat surprising, but the use of the two different words probably was intended to guard against a literalistic material misinterpretation: The "image" is of a particular kind, namely, a *likeness* or *reflection,* not a physical representation.

What exactly is reflected–that is, the exact meaning of this concept–has been hotly debated for millennia, and it is far beyond the scope of this brief article to enter the debate. It seems indisputable, though, that the clear intention of the story is to convey the uniqueness of human beings and their relationship to their Creator when compared to all other living beings, none of which shares this likeness (though they do share other characteristics, like mode of creation, for instance). Many contemporary scholars conclude, for example, that the real purpose of this language was to suggest that human beings serve as God's "representatives" on earth in the same way that statues of kings reminded inhabitants of their rulers (cf. the fact that God explicitly grants humans "dominion" over all the earth in Genesis 1:28, an authority conveyed in Genesis 2:19 in the other creation story's more poetic style by the man's naming of all the animals). The point is that whatever the precise meaning of the image of God in which humans are created, such creation clearly confers upon them uniqueness and dignity by virtue of a special relationship with God and their preeminent place of authority in the created order (cf. Psalm 8:5-6: "Yet you have made them a little lower than God, and crowned them with glory and honor. You have given them dominion over the works of your hands; you have put all things under their feet.").

Here we see already the importance of recognizing that where we stand colors what we see. More will be said later about the implications of this doctrine for pastoral care; at this point, though, it is interesting to note that the understanding of the "image of God" that seems most popular today (not surprisingly given our post-Enlightenment emphasis on rationality) is that it refers to our ability to reason, to produce complex language, or to relate to one another and to God in ways mediated by our intellect. Clearly, this interpretation creates problems for persons with dementia, in which all of these capacities are precisely the ones that are lost. The less specific view expressed above, however–that creation in the image of God simply gives to human beings a uniqueness that confers special dignity and worth upon them–opens up possibilities (and obligations) for care of even those whose cognitive function is greatly diminished.

THE PSYCHOPHYSICAL NATURE OF HUMAN BEINGS

A second and closely related aspect of ancient Hebrew anthropology is also instructive in this context, although unfortunately it too has suffered in later Christian thought, primarily through the infiltration of Greek values. Interestingly, however, this idea is currently enjoying a resurgence of acceptance based on the findings of modern scientific medicine. I am speaking of what has been called the concept of the human being as a *psychophysical* or *psychosomatic unity*.

For the early Hebrews, the "body" and "soul" or "flesh" and "spirit" were not separate entities that just accidentally (or even evilly) came to be joined in some way; instead, they were seen as interdependent elements that are both necessary for a human being to exist. The term often translated *soul* in the creation accounts of Genesis, *nephesh*, really means something more like *life-force, life-principle*, or simply *vitality*. When it "goes out" (in the sense of departing), the individual ceases to exist (a claim corroborated, incidentally, by the lack of any concept of personal, individual immortality in Hebrew religion, at least until the post-exilic period–cf. Jesus' debate with the Sadducees, Matthew 22:23; also Acts 23:8). Thus the mental and physical activities of an individual are merely different manifestations of the same underlying living being. Instead of *having* a body, as we tend today to think of ourselves, as if the *real* person is somehow separate from the body, the person in fact *is* a body. The human being in short is both an animated body and an incarnate soul, or, as the late ethicist Paul Ramsey (1970, 87) so aptly expressed it, "the body of his soul no less than . . . the soul (mind, will) of his body."

This concept is admittedly very difficult for those in the Greek-influenced, Cartesian thought-world we inhabit, with its dualistic view that separates human nature into a material body and some kind of "spiritual" entity that outlives (and truth be told, "outvalues") the body. Some will also argue that the Christian faith has moved beyond this ancient Hebrew view to one that does in fact affirm an immortal soul as a separate entity. Indeed, most Christians are so thoroughly imbued with dualistic values that they lose sight of the fact that what they actually affirm as their belief about eternal life is *not* the Greek "immortality of the *soul*" but the much more Hebraic notion of the "resurrection of the *body*"! Before moving on to consider several other biblical ideas relevant to our topic, therefore, it may be wise to pause and see how these first two can help us "see things as God sees them" in an effort to find guidance in providing pastoral care to persons with dementia.

Because of the discomfort of later Christian tradition with the material aspects of creation (*all* of which, we need constantly to remind ourselves, receive in Genesis 1:31 the assessment "very good" from their Creator), the image of God was initially spiritualized (i.e., interpreted as referring to the capacity to make moral decisions, e.g., or to relate to God in a deliberate, conscious way) and more recently intellectualized (i.e., understood as reflecting the ability to reason or to engage in complex cognition and language). Similarly, the psychophysical unity of human nature was sundered at first in the direction of an overemphasis on spirit and a consequent devaluation of the body (e.g., in the monastic tradition), followed by a move toward the denial of everything *but* the material aspects (as in Freudian and other reductionistic theories), and now once again a shift toward a denigration of the body in favor of the "rational" or "cognitive" dimension (as in contemporary attempts to redefine "humanhood" to require higher-brain function). The moves within theological anthropology thus have meshed perfectly with more secular forces to lead to what Stephen Post (1995) has aptly labeled our "hypercognitive culture."

Such a society, born of Enlightenment rationalism, values clarity of thought and the ability to perform complex cognitive operations as the sources of human dignity and worth and is quite content to dismiss as useless (if even human) those who no longer possess such capacities (or never did). Clearly, persons suffering from dementia such as AD–which takes from them precisely that which our society increasingly sees as giving human beings value, in fact, as making us *human,* namely, our memory, reason, and language and thus our ability to be "productive and contributing" members of society–are prime candidates to be devalued, to be considered less than fully human, perhaps even to be called "vegetables" and therefore not treated with the respect we still at least affirm is due all human beings.

In addition to being a product of Enlightenment rationalism, our culture is also deeply rooted in capitalism as well. Indeed, it is hard to decide which influence predominates, and perhaps it is therefore safest to say simply that if Americans believe that there is anything that confers worth to a person more than *rationality,* it is *productivity.*[3] And that productivity is almost always measured in economic terms, which creates immediate problems for the elderly in general and those with dementia in particular. As someone has said, the American paradox is to glory in individualism but to value the individual chiefly for what s/he achieves in society. It is not hard to determine what such a society's opinion will be of someone who is judged to have lost both individuality and productivity to dementia.

Sadly, I have detected even among many people of faith–and I do not exclude myself–a disposition to buy into this view. We increasingly accept the "self-evident" proposition that a person who does not think is less than fully human (if even that), that someone who is no longer "productive" is not really a person, in short, that the inherent value that we have heretofore automatically attributed to humans as beings created in God's own image is unquestionably lost or certainly diminished by the loss of rationality and economic productivity.

There can be little question that our society needs to give this shift in our fundamental understanding of human nature much more serious attention than we have so far, and dementia is certainly a logical framework within which to do that. Those who stand in one of our historic faith traditions must be part of this debate and–acknowledging the difficulties raised by our traditional understanding (and frequent *mis*understanding) of church-state relations–at least make an effort to ensure that this country continue to see all persons as God sees them. Over the past several decades, for example, many faithful people have questioned the values of our consumer society that affirm, in Erich Fromm's (1976, 15) words, that "I am = what I have and what I consume." And the conclusion in this "being vs. *having*" conflict has been overwhelmingly that the biblical religions come down firmly on the side of being over having as the criterion for human worth. To see things as God sees them suggests that it is now incumbent upon us to confront our hypercognitive society's move toward the claim that "I am = my ability to think" (which is actually merely a modern reaffirmation of the 17th-century French philosopher René Descartes' famous dictum *Cogito ergo sum*–"I think, therefore I am"). As we now begin to address the "being vs. *thinking*" conflict, a careful study of our historical texts and traditions–enlightened by the best of modern knowledge–can contribute a great deal to protecting those whose ability to protect themselves is limited, as such study has done many times in the past.

I would suggest that given the emphasis in the biblical creation accounts on the goodness of the material aspects of that creation, coupled with these stories' presentation of the nature of human beings outlined above, it is likely that if we truly are concerned with seeing things as God sees them, we need to rethink some of the basic assumptions gaining favor today about what it is that gives human beings value. It is logical to assume that as God looks upon those created in God's own image (even if that image is less than God originally intended–and Christian theology certainly asserts that sin has brought about that diminished condition in *every* human being, however rational or cognitively intact), God sees a being by definition worthy of respect and consideration because in some sense God sees God's reflection there.[4]

DEPENDENCE

The discussion of our hypercognitive culture's emphasis on a fully working brain and economic productivity as the source of human worth and dignity leads quite naturally into another important facet of the concerns this article addresses and suggests another central tenet of biblical religion that says a great deal to us about pastoral care to persons with AD. The only personal characteristic that comes readily to mind that our society values more highly than cognitive functioning is the "A-word"–*autonomy*. If one thing terrifies Americans more than the thought of losing their minds, it is the thought of losing their independence (the two are of course closely linked). As William F. May (1982, 32) so aptly puts it, "Americans have historically taken pride in themselves as an independent people. . . . The dark side of this aspiration to self-reliance is an abhorrence of dependency." Anyone who has ever had to deal with an elderly person concerning the matter of "the car keys" (a common problem for caregivers of people with dementia) understands only too well what May is talking about, and this obsession with independence permeates the very fiber of our culture. Unfortunately, just as dementia inexorably leads to the loss of cognitive function, so it also unavoidably brings on that "abhorrent" condition of dependence.

What does theology have to offer in this situation? Again, quite a bit, though here also space limitations permit only the barest outline. The western religious tradition asserts unanimously that the *normal* (and proper) human condition *is* one of dependence, though each religion expresses this fact differently. For its part, Christianity is at its very heart all about being dependent, accepting the fact that one does not live on one's own and only for oneself at *any* point in one's life, not just when one must face the losses of dementia (or, one might add, of even so-called "healthy" aging). If one accepts the central Christian doctrine that the death of Jesus Christ alone is sufficient to restore the broken relationship between human beings and their Creator, then one must acknowledge one's absolute dependence on the unmerited and freely given grace of God. The Apostle Paul puts it in about as "non-independent" language as it can be put when he says, "It is no longer I who live, but Christ who lives in me" (Galatians 2:20), hardly a view with which most Americans today are comfortable. We want instead to be "our own person," to "do our own thing," to "make it on our own." But accepting the totally free grace of God as the condition for salvation is nothing less than acknowledging utter and ultimate dependence upon God.

If we refuse to admit dependence, however, we cannot really express gratitude, to God or to our fellow human beings, and we tend therefore to concentrate instead on *rights* as a way of escaping the admission of our own dependence: That is, if what I am receiving from you is my *right,* then I am not really dependent on you for it, nor do I have to thank you for giving it to me. I *deserve* it. If, on the other hand, we can acknowledge that we are totally dependent throughout our lives on the creating, redeeming, and sustaining God, then perhaps it will be easier to accept increasing dependence upon other human beings as we age and face the infirmities that accompany it. At any rate, if we try to see others as God sees us, then we will be careful about devaluing them because of their lost independence out of our realization that in God's eyes, we are just as dependent as they are–on the scale that really matters.

One further aspect of this cardinal belief merits mention before moving on. In Romans 3:22*b*-24, Paul states clearly the theological foundation upon which his teachings rest: "For there is no distinction, since all have sinned and fall short of the glory of God; they are now justified by his grace as a gift, through the redemption that is in Christ Jesus." Thus no one can claim superiority over anyone else–any more on the basis of better cognitive function than on other grounds like race, wealth, or supposed greater moral virtue–because all stand on the common ground of having been redeemed from sin by the death of Jesus Christ. In this way Paul expands the equality of all human beings implied by their shared creation "in the image of God" to include a distinctively Christian element. As being created in God's likeness gives dignity and worth to all human beings, so also (and even more so) does the willingness of God's Son to die for them.

COMMUNITY (MEMBERS OF THE "BODY")

Another basic concept in Christianity that can be helpful in this discussion is the importance of community, expressed especially vividly in Paul's image of the church as the body of Christ (echoing in many ways Judaism's notion of the covenant people). It is clear from what has already been said that, in contrast to the radically individualistic attitude espoused by contemporary American society, our dominant religious traditions strongly affirm that human beings are *more* than merely autonomous beings who exist as separate atoms in discrete moments of time, able to do exactly as they please whenever they please. The biblical religions assert in ways too numerous even to mention here that God sees humans not as such radically disconnected individuals but as *social-historical* beings who are undeniably linked with others, living in community and changing over time in ways over which they do not always have control. These conditions necessarily limit our autonomy and make clear the naiveté of interpreting it as absolute freedom to choose whatever we want whenever we want. Indeed, ethicist Lisa Sowle Cahill (1985, 152) claims that "the horizon against which *all* moral activity is to be evaluated is the communal life as body of Christ in the world."

What exactly does this intriguing metaphor mean? Among many instructive lessons, let me mention only two that seem most relevant to the concerns of this article, drawing on Paul's presentation in I Corinthians 12. First, if we relate to one another as members of one body, beyond the obvious fact that we will in general be more tolerant of others, we should also more readily recognize that the suffering or injury of one member necessarily has an impact on all the others. Whatever can be done to prevent or alleviate suffering for any member, then, will benefit both every other member and the body as a whole: "If one member suffers, all suffer together with it; if one member is honored, all rejoice together with it" (v. 26). Second, Paul goes on to make the interesting point that this organic union also means that the "more presentable" members have no basis for denigrating or neglecting those who are "less honorable." Indeed, he goes so far as to say that "the members of the body that seem to be weaker are indispensable" (v. 22) and that "God has so arranged the body, giving the *greater* honor to the *inferior* member, that there may be no dissension within the body, but the members may have the same care for one another" (vv. 24-25, emphasis added). The implications for seeing demented persons as God sees them–at least within Christian "bodies"–hardly need to be made explicit here.

One further thought arises before leaving this point. It is interesting in this context to play a word game with the word *remember*–so central in any discussion of dementia–by inserting a hyphen in it: *re-member*. As people lose their cognitive capacities in our hypercognitive society, they tend to be shunted to the periphery, to have their very "humanhood" questioned, certainly to be treated with less than the full dignity that we have seen our dominant religious traditions ascribe to every human being. But if the community of faith–the "body" of which they are an organic part–*remembers* them by continuing to treat them like those whom God sees as beloved children, then in a very real sense that community will be *re-membering* those individuals in the sense of bringing them back into the human community, refusing to let them be cast aside and forgotten, which is in effect to *dis*-member the body. And chaplains are often in an especially critical position to facilitate this process of re-membering as individuals are removed from their normal environment into health care institutions of various kinds.

GOD'S DIFFERENT STANDARDS

If the goal of chaplains responsible for pastoral care to persons with dementia is as much as possible to see things as God sees them, the

Apostle Paul once more speaks very clearly on this issue in I Corinthians 1:18-31, especially vv. 26-29. In a nutshell, Paul asserts that acceptance of the Christian gospel does not require of a person great intelligence or wisdom, nor is it something that can be bought by great wealth (interestingly, Paul alludes here to the two values contemporary American society holds most dear: cognitive functioning and economic status). The basis for his view is of course the heart of the gospel already mentioned above, namely, that salvation cannot be gained on one's own by *any* means but requires merely the acceptance of God's freely offered grace. In order to make this clear, Paul points out how God has chosen those who are weak and foolish "according to worldly standards" as the vehicle of redemption, precisely in order to show the insignificance of the "wisdom of the wise and the cleverness of the clever." His point is unmistakable: God judges by standards that differ markedly from those of the world.

Granted, the Apostle does not refer explicitly to persons with dementia (or even to the elderly), but given the attitude that is developing in our society toward such people and their worth, it does not seem unfair to apply Paul's affirmations in this passage to them as well. The world still values those who are "wise," "powerful," and "of noble birth," but as I have argued, added to the list today are the "cognitively functional," the "relationally capable," the "economically productive," and the "able-bodied" (though the sage and sobering warning of Daniel Callahan is worth noting here, that those of us who think *we* have just been described should remember that the word "currently" properly belongs in front of each of those phrases!). If, however, as Paul makes clear in this passage, God sees things so very differently from the way the world does–and judges by such different, even diametrically opposed, standards–we had best be very careful in our evaluations of those whose cognitive and relational capacities are diminished by dementia.

SOME PRACTICAL APPLICATIONS

I have suggested throughout this look at basic theological concepts some ways that they can inform pastoral care of people suffering from dementia. Clearly, underlying any approach to meeting the spiritual needs of such people must be a lively respect for their ongoing dignity and worth as human beings, as those whom God has created and values as any parent does a child, even if that child is not perfect. I want now to present in summary form one way that has been suggested for structuring pastoral care for people with dementia and their caregivers.[5] Because of space limitations, I cannot describe the approach in detail, but as we look at its components, their grounding in the theological doctrines outlined above will be clear. Indeed, the very model itself–using the acrostic *DIGNITY*–speaks vividly to the fundamental goal of caring for individuals with dementia.

D: Draw out the person's (and family's) past. Even if the person can no longer remember, he or she *does* have a unique history that deserves to be considered. Discover that uniqueness, including religious/ cultural factors, and respond accordingly. One important role of the faith community can be to remember *for* the person when she or he can no longer do so.

I: Individualize the intervention. As Alzheimer's caregivers are fond of saying, "When you've seen one person with Alzheimer's . . . you've seen one person with Alzheimer's." Some respond to familiar scripture passages or old hymns, others to familiar rituals or symbols of the faith. Realize also that the same person may be different from visit to visit and deal with the person you find. But always keep in mind that this is a unique individual who deserves your best effort to provide care in a way that is personally meaningful to him or her.

G: God's plan is paramount. Chaplains are not there to cure or to fix but to embody God's presence in whatever ways they can devise. Expect frustration and feelings of helplessness, perhaps even anger sometimes, but remember that in God's eyes all humans are impaired, just in different ways. Accept the advice offered by Donna Cohen and Carl Eisdorfer (1986, 193), two of the leading researchers in the field, that "a key to coping successfully is to recognize that the caregiver role is impossible and then to try to do the best you can" (I would add, "and leave the outcome to God"). Above all, chaplains need to keep firmly in mind that even Superman is Clark Kent most of the time!

N: Needs of the patient and family caregivers must be kept foremost in any pastoral care plan. Remember that just because the person seems unable to function cognitively does not mean that he or she is of no value and no longer has spiritual needs; try to maintain a holistic view, honoring the body that has been the channel and vehicle for the now-lost intellectual operations and memories. Also, do not *over*estimate the needs of patient or family; as Marty Richards, a geriatric social worker in Seattle with three decades of experience in the field, is fond of saying, "When our need to help is stronger than the need to be helped, help strikes again!"

I: Informed intervention is essential. That is, learn all you can about dementia and the effect it has on patients and caregivers, through every avenue available to you. As Henry Simmons and Mark Peters (1996, 56) point out, "We can offer no better advice to a first-time visitor . . . than to ask for help and orientation (at a time negotiated with the staff)." Knowing when to ask for help or to refer a patient or family member to someone more experienced or better trained is also important.

T: Turn down your pace; expect delays; be patient. Depending on the level of impairment of the person with dementia, visits may be quite lengthy as efforts are made to communicate–often in novel ways –or quite brief as no form of intervention reaches the person (though prayer is always appropriate in such cases unless it has been explicitly ruled out in some way). Remember that God may see the person very differently from the way we do. Simmons and Peters (1996, 57) again offer wise counsel: "Time lovingly spent in attentive, loving presence or a shared pleasure is a precious gift."

Y: Your preparation is critical. Before visiting a person with dementia, be sure to pray for humility, wisdom, discernment, strength, and a lively sense of both perspective and humor. Reflect on the theological concepts discussed above in light of your own faith tradition's exposition of them and consider ways you might apply them to your own attitude toward and interaction with those who suffer from an illness that takes from them all those characteristics our society says gives them value.

Informing each aspect of this model is a genuine attempt to see persons with dementia as God sees them, a lively awareness of the continuing reflection of God in them and of their ongoing value even if they are no longer able to function cognitively. This approach evaluates such people by standards quite different from those dominant in the larger society and recognizes that through the efforts of chaplains and others in the faith community such persons can remain members of that community despite their inability to participate in normal ways.

THE IMPORTANCE OF CHAPLAINS

I want to conclude with just a couple more personal comments to those who are "in the trenches" day in and day out, providing pastoral care to vulnerable people, whether those with dementia or some other affliction. The first thing I have to say to you is that I have discovered in my own work–not just with older people but in any area in which I have hoped that my efforts might in some way make this messy world a little better place for us all to live–that it is easy to get discouraged and ask in despair, "What's the point? I can't possibly hope to change things." If you ever find yourself feeling that way–and in any kind of confrontation with AD it is not an unreasonable way to feel–please remember a magnificent statement made by the poet-statesman Vaclav Havel: "Hope is not about believing you can change things. Hope is about believing you make a difference." Trust me: Chaplains make a difference. As a patient noted about the role her faith played in her terminal illness, "Hope is not to believe that I will be cured but that even if I am not, God will be there with me throughout whatever I face." The chaplain is one of the most visible and potentially meaningful expressions of God's presence in health care institutions.

If discouragement ever takes the form of saying, "I'm not so sure I even make much of a difference, remember this story. A man, out for a walk on the beach early one morning, noticed a lone figure far down the beach repeatedly bending over, picking something up, and throwing it out into the water. Intrigued, he quickened his pace and soon came close enough to see it was an old man. He asked the man what he was doing, and he replied, "You see all these starfish. When the tide comes in it washes them ashore, and then the tide goes out and they can't get back to the water. When the sun comes up, they die. So I'm throwing them back." My friend was touched by the old man's compassion but he couldn't help chuckling to himself and saying to the man, "That is very kind of you, but there must be hundreds of starfish right here, and hundreds of miles of beach. What possible difference do you think you, just one person, can make to all these starfish?" The old man looked him in the eye, bent over and picked up another starfish, and flung it out into the surf. Continuing to gaze at the ripples, he said quietly, "Made a difference to that one."[6]

NOTES

1. An excellent source that provides a broad overview as well as much specific information in this regard is Koenig, 1994.

2. Much fuller treatment of the concepts discussed below can be found in several of the books listed in the References. The *Journal of Religious Gerontology,* also

published by The Haworth Press, Inc., is another source for timely and relevant articles. Sapp (1996) is an accessible guidebook for clergy and families describing the impact of Alzheimer's Disease that many family caregivers especially have reported to be very helpful. It is available free from Desert Ministries, P.O. Box 788, Palm Beach, FL 33480. The Forum on Religion, Spirituality, and Aging (FoRSA) of the American Society on Aging (415-974-9600) sponsors sessions at ASA's annual meeting each March and its Summer Series in various major cities that provide useful information and give participants opportunities to meet and interact with others who are interested in providing the best care possible to aging persons. And a resource that should always be kept in mind is the national Alzheimer's Association (1-800-272-3900), a source for both the latest research about Alzheimer's and, perhaps even more important, the phone number of the nearest local chapter.

3. The two values are of course closely if not inextricably interrelated–philosophically, historically, and certainly practically (though I would seriously question the rationality of some people that our popular culture considers among its most productive).

4. I have explored several of these issues more fully in Sapp (1998). That article is an excerpt from one of two chapters I contributed to McKim (1997), which contain even more complete discussions.

6. This model was presented by Jon C. Stuckey, PhD (Senior Research Associate, University Alzheimer Center, Case Western Reserve University/University Hospitals of Cleveland) at a workshop titled "Finding Meaning in Dementia Caregiving," in San Francisco on March 25, 1998. The workshop was part of the 1998 FoRSA special program, "Reasons to Grow Old: Charting a Course to Value and Meaning" mentioned in Note 1 above.

6. Adapted from Canfield and Hansen (1993, 22-23).

REFERENCES

Cahill, L. (1985). *Between the Sexes: Foundations for a Christian Ethics of Sexuality.* Philadelphia: Fortress Press; New York: Paulist Press.

Canfield, J., Hansen, M. (1993). *Chicken Soup for the Soul: 101 Stories to Open the Heart and Rekindle the Spirit.* Deerfield Beach, Florida: Health Communications, Inc.

Cohen, D., Eisdorfer, C. (1986). *The Loss of Self: A Family Resource for the Care of Alzheimer's Disease and Related Disorders.* New York: W. W. Norton.

Fromm, E. (1976). *To Be or To Have?* New York: Bantam Books.

Keck, D. (1996). *Forgetting Whose We Are: Alzheimer's Disease and the Love of God.* Nashville: Abingdon Press.

Koenig, H. (1994). *Aging and God: Spiritual Pathways to Mental Health in Midlife and Later Years.* New York: The Haworth Pastoral Press.

McKim, D., ed. (1997). *God Never Forgets: Faith, Hope, and Alzheimer's Disease.* Louisville: Westminster John Knox Press.

May, W. (1982). Who cares for the elderly? *Hastings Center Report,* 12 (December 1982), 31-37.

Post, S. (1995). *The Moral Challenge of Alzheimer Disease*. Baltimore: Johns Hopkins University Press.

Ramsey, P. (1970). *Fabricated Man: The Ethics of Genetic Control*. New Haven: Yale University Press.

Sapp, S. (1996). *When Alzheimer's Disease Strikes*. Palm Beach, FL: Desert Ministries.

Sapp, S. (1998). Living with Alzheimer's: Body, soul and the remembering community. *Christian Century,* 115, 2 (January 21, 1998), 54-60.

Simmons, H., Peters, M. (1996). *With God's Oldest Friends: Pastoral Visiting in the Nursing Home*. New York: Paulist Press.

Spirituality, Religion, and Alzheimer's Disease

Stephen G. Post, PhD
Peter J. Whitehouse, MD, PhD

SUMMARY. The chaplain's ministry to persons with dementia, often of the Alzheimer's type, is vitally relevant to their clinical well-being. No chaplain should even think that because someone is demented, they can no longer be reached spiritually. While few scientific studies exist, clinical experience and anecdotal accounts suggest that selected pastoral interventions can enhance the quality of life of the mildly, moderately, and even severely demented individual. *[Article copies available for a fee from The Haworth Document Delivery Service: 1-800-342-9678. E-mail address: getinfo@haworthpressinc.com]*

Chaplains can engage Alzheimer's disease (AD) victims in a clinically relevant ministry. On some occasions, chaplains might think, "I need not provide ministry to this person because s/he won't remember anything anyway." However, persons possess more than memory and intellect; they also have emotion, relationship, imagination, will, and aesthetic awareness. As Chaplain Debbie Everett (1997) said at a national meeting of the U.S. Alzheimer's Association:

> If a deeper experience of life could be realized by myself through a greater awareness of touch, music, human presence, love,

---

Stephen G. Post is affiliated with the Center for Biomedical Ethics, Department of Religion and Peter J. Whitehouse is Director, University Alzheimer Center, Center for Biomedical Ethics, both at Case Western Reserve University, Cleveland, OH.

[Haworth co-indexing entry note]: "Spirituality, Religion, and Alzheimer's Disease." Post, Stephen G., and Peter J. Whitehouse. Co-published simultaneously in *Journal of Health Care Chaplaincy* (The Haworth Pastoral Press, an imprint of The Haworth Press, Inc.) Vol. 8, No. 1/2, 1999, pp. 45-57; and: *Spiritual Care for Persons with Dementia: Fundamentals for Pastoral Practice* (ed: Larry VandeCreek) The Haworth Pastoral Press, an imprint of The Haworth Press, Inc., 1999, pp. 45-57. Single or multiple copies of this article are available for a fee from The Haworth Document Delivery Service [1-800-342-9678, 9:00 a.m. - 5:00 p.m. (EST). E-mail address: getinfo@haworthpressinc.com].

45

smell, color, play, laughter, nature and so on, what could this mean in the lives of those with Alzheimer's disease? In discovering how to better meet the spiritual needs of these people, in essence I found what spirituality means in a wider context beyond intellect, in the realm of our bodies and emotions.

Everett notes that spirituality in eastern and western religions includes an awareness of the present moment; from that perspective individuals with AD may even teach us something. She writes, "The paradigm shift that I advocate in the care of those affected by AD is to discover and appreciate a wider range of communication possibilities."

Oliver Sacks' (1970) compelling description of a patient with a severe Korsakov's dementia makes the same point.

> Seeing Jim in the chapel opened my eyes to other realms where the soul is called on, and held, and stilled, in attention and communion. The same depth of absorption and attention was to be seen in relation to music and art: he had no difficultly. (p. 38)

Sacks continues:

> But if he was held in emotional and spiritual attention–in the contemplation of nature or art, in listening to music, in taking part in the Mass in chapel–the attention, its "mood," its quietude, would persist for a while, and there would be in him a pensiveness and peace we rarely, if ever saw during the rest of his life . . . . (p. 39)

Despite the confusion of dementia, Sacks points out "the undiminished possibility of reintegration by art, by communion, by touching the human spirit: and this can be preserved in what seems at first a hopeless state of neurological devastation" (p. 38).

The observations of Everett and Sacks are not surprising. The clinical evidence for the impact of religion and spirituality on many areas related to health and illness has increased steadily, including health enhancement, coping with illness, as well as prevention of suicide, depression, substance abuse, heart disease, and high blood pressure. Mounting empirical studies demonstrate that for many Americans, religious beliefs and practices are a very important means of coping with major illness (Larson and Milano 1995). It is reasonable to mount research projects concerning the impact of spirituality and pastoral care on dementia, the contemporary epidemic. Such clinical studies likely will be helpful although they are slow to emerge partly because of research methodological problems.

Having suggested, even insisted, that pastoral care of persons with AD is relevant and that they merit spiritual attention, it is necessary to note that clinicians in Western medicine place a Jeffersonian wall of separation between the spheres of medical practice and attention to the individual's religion and spirituality. This as well as overwhelming attention to empirical medicine has blinded many clinicians to the importance of spiritual and religious concerns in the medical condition. Presently, this wall is being replaced by a fence, a positive development because fences "make good neighbors" by allowing both conversations and boundaries. Such conversations can lead to increased recognition of spiritual needs of persons and the importance of pastoral care. However, all parties, including chaplains, physicians, and administrators have obligations here. Chaplains need to remember that a major continuing impediment for physicians who wish to refer AD individuals for spiritual attention is the concern that religion will be imposed on vulnerable individuals. All the negative stereotypes associated with "preachers" can be exceptionally influential and prevent such referrals. In turn, physicians and administrators must recognize that the best antidote to this concern is the chaplain's participation in accredited clinical pastoral education experiences. Administrators create significant professional barriers when they employ untrained and/insensitive clergy to provide pastoral care to persons with dementia.

An additional way to clarify these concerns for the skeptical physician or administrator is to point out the difference between spirituality and religion. Spirituality, in contrast to religion, pertains to a sense of relatedness to nature, all humanity, and the Transcendent. Although it need not be the case, spirituality often is contextualized within a religious tradition, i.e., a specific system of belief, worship, and conduct. Given persons with increasing dementia, attention to doctrine, dogma, and beliefs are ill advised in this ministry if they require cognitive function and memory.

We now address a more personal question as regards AD. How might a person find meaning and a degree of inner peace when informed of an AD diagnosis? The person must navigate a journey into deep forgetfulness that only seems slightly less anxious when one forgets that one forgets. Caregivers, in turn, may be shaken to their spiritual foundations by unexpected responsibilities. Spirituality in AD refers to essential meanings, including theological ones, that shape experience and create attitudes of hope, trust, courage, perseverance, and other ways of being-in-the-world for both the AD-affected person and caregivers.

In the remainder of this article, we apply questions of spirituality and religion directly to the context of the care of people with AD. Additional scientific research on interventions and outcomes in quality of life is required before chaplains can know with clarity exactly what they should be doing with and for people with AD at its various stages. Even without data, however, chaplains need to realize their clinical relevance in enhancing quality of life for persons with dementia and their caregivers.

SPIRITUALITY AND AD PREVENTION?

Does spirituality have a role in AD prevention? Some people with AD live for two decades after initial clinical symptoms, although most live for no more than seven or eight years. Prevalence of the disease doubles every five years after age 65, when an estimated 3 percent of individuals are affected, to reach at least one third of those 85 years of age or older (the so-called "old-old"). There may be a plateau affect after the ninth decade of life, so that an estimated 2 of 3 people among the "old-old" will remain free of AD, although this point of view remains controversial. Four million Americans now suffer with AD; a projected 12 million will in 2050 (Canada will approach 1 million), absent cure or prevention. This specter may be mitigated by emerging preventive technologies such as estrogen and Vitamin E, both still under investigation, linked with more refined susceptibility tests.

Some (Sapolsky 1992; Lupien et al. 1994) suggest spirituality as a preventive approach to AD. This is based on studies of cognitive dysfunction in rats brought on by stress-related elevation of catecholamines and serum cortisol which are toxic to neurons. The meditative relaxation response, already widely prescribed for patients with hypertension, chronic pain, and other ailments, could conceivably impact memory retention, although this is purely hypothetical and has not yet been studied scientifically (Khalsa 1996).

Thus, it would come as no surprise to the authors if evidence uncovered in the future indicates that the moral and spiritual tone of a person's earlier life shapes behavior in the demented condition to a greater or lesser degree. Chaplains need to be aware that their spiritual work among currently healthy individuals may have some future neurological and/or behavioral impact relevant to AD.

SPIRITUALITY AND DIAGNOSTIC DISCLOSURE

Chaplains have a significant role in the disclosure of a diagnosis as serious as AD. They encourage hope despite the future perils of forgetfulness. Hope is a multidimensional dynamic attribute that concerns dimensions of possibility and confidence in the future (Frankl 1963). Hope can address secular matters such as future plans and relationships, or religious matters of ultimate destiny. Hope is an aspect of "spiritual" well-being. Many studies concerning hope exist in the nursing literature, usually pertaining to cancer patients and those with AIDS. Increasing attention must be given to the role of hope with those suffering from AD.

Preservation of hope can maximize psychological adjustment to a severe dementia. The importance of a spirituality of hope in the lives of people with disability has been summarized at the Conference on "The Roles of Religiousness and Spirituality in Rehabilitation and the Lives of those with Disability," held at the National Institutes of Health in May, 1995 (Underwood-Gordon 1995). Hope need not exist within the context of a world religion, although it often does.

Although only indirectly relevant to AD, a 1993 survey conducted in an inpatient rehabilitation unit indicated that 74% of patients hold their religious and spiritual beliefs to be important, 54% desire pastoral counseling, and 45% think not enough attention is given to the spiritual and religious beliefs. The authors concluded that rehabilitation personnel should be aware of the diversity of religious beliefs held by patients, and should address these when necessary with respect (Anderson et al., 1993).

Hope is the subjective sense of having a meaningful future despite obstacles. In times of severe disabling injury, hope may be mediated through ritual, meditation, prayer, and traditional sacred narratives. Many experience hope in the context of a spiritual-religious construct.

Ethically, the disclosure of a diagnosis of probable AD allows the person to plan for the best use of remaining years of mental capacity, to participate actively in support groups, to consider consenting for AD research projects, and to make known preferences for future levels of medical treatment after the dementia becomes severe. Yet some clinicians still resist telling the patient about his or her diagnosis, often because they do not wish to create despair. But in the effort to retain hope, the whole ethical process of looking toward future choices is undone.

Active pastoral care in the clinical context of diagnosis could encourage the retention of hope during and after diagnostic disclosure. The following questions are relevant to the clinical context (Maugens 1996):

- How do you think your dementia will affect your life?
- Who or what helps you to keep a positive outlook about life in spite of your dementia?
- Is there any way in which dementia itself has caused positive changes for you?
- What is the most difficult thing about your dementia?
- Have you been discouraged or depressed about your dementia? When?
- When you feel yourself getting discouraged, how do you pull your spirits back up?
- Are there family members who are especially helpful? Who and how do they help?
- Do you believe there is a reason or purpose for your dementia? If yes, what do you think that reason or purpose is?
- Do you think that your religious beliefs and community can contribute to your well-being in these circumstances?

Such a spiritual history and inventory can be very useful in understanding their sources of well-being, and in helping them to identify spiritual resources in the community. Clinicians should acknowledge the importance of spirituality and religion in diagnosed individuals, refer to clergy, but also readily respond to spirituality concerns as these arise.

SPIRITUALITY AND QUALITY OF LIFE
IN DIAGNOSED INDIVIDUALS

One of the finest autobiographical accounts of living with the diagnosis and initial decline of AD is *My Journey into Alzheimer's Disease* by Rev. Robert Davis (1989). He writes as follows:

> One night in Wyoming, as I lay in a motel crying out to my Lord, my long desperate prayers were suddenly answered. As I lay there in the blackness silently shrieking out my often repeated prayer, there was suddenly a light that seemed to fill my very soul. The sweet, holy presence of Christ came to me. He spoke to my spirit and said, "Take my peace. Stop your struggling. It is all right. This is all in keeping with my will for your life. . . . Lie back in your Shepherd's arms, and take my peace." (p. 55)

As Rev. Davis "mourned the loss of old abilities," he nevertheless could draw on his religious faith: "I choose to take things moment by moment, thankful for everything that I have, instead of raging wildly at the things that I have lost" (p. 57). Yet as he struggled to find a degree of peace amidst decline, he was also keenly aware of people who "simply cannot handle being around someone who is mentally and emotionally impaired" (p. 115). In his church community, and through the love of his wife, the journey was at least more navigable.

People with a diagnosis of AD often pray, for they are thrown back onto whatever faith they have in the meaningful and beneficent purposes underlying the universe. They pray because the routine and the control has been taken from their lives, and probably because they fear the future. They are shaken existentially, and must begin a final phase of their journey in remarkable trust. The person with a diagnosis of AD will often desire to pray with family members, to pray in religious communities, and to pray alone. The word prayer comes from the Latin *precari,* "to entreat," or ask earnestly. It comes from the same root as the word precarious, and it is in the precariousness of emerging forgetfulness that often the person with dementia is driven to prayer. Prayer is one way of enhancing hope in the future despite dementia. Chaplains and clinicians should encourage this propensity to gain strength through prayer in the midst of cognitive decline.

To present the picture of people with dementia as meaning seeking, we borrow from an autobiographical account in Post's book, *The*

Moral Challenge of Alzheimer Disease (1995). The following story–only lightly edited–was told by a woman in her mid-40's with dementia, etiology unknown. She is conversant, although there are some days when she is too mentally confused to engage in much dialogue. She has more difficulty responding to open-ended questions, but does very well if her conversation partner cues her by mentioning several alternative words from which she might choose, at which point she can be quite articulate.

It was just about this time three years ago that I recall laughing with my sister while in dance class at my turning the big 40. "Don't worry, life begins at forty," she exclaimed and then sweetly advised her younger sister of all the wonders in life still to be found. Little did either of us realize what a cruel twist life was proceeding to take. It was a fate neither she nor I ever imagined someone in our age group could encounter.

Things began to happen that I just couldn't understand. There were times I addressed friends by the wrong name. Comprehending conversations seemed almost impossible. My attention span became quite short. Notes were needed to remind me of things to be done and how to do them. I would slur my speech, use inappropriate words, or simply eliminate one from a sentence. This caused not only frustration for me but also a great deal of embarrassment. Then came the times I honestly could not remember how to plan a meal or shop for groceries.

One day, while out for a walk on my usual path in a city in which I had resided for 11 years, nothing looked familiar. It was as if I was lost in a foreign land, yet I had the sense to ask for directions home.

There were more days than not when I was perfectly fine; but to me, they did not make up for the ones that weren't. I knew there was something terribly wrong and after 18 months of undergoing a tremendous amount of tests and countless visits to various doctors, I was proven right.

Dementia is the disease, they say, cause unknown. At this point it no longer mattered to me just what that cause was because the tests eliminated the reversible ones, my hospital coverage was gone, and my spirit was too worn to even care about the name of something irreversible.

I was angry. I was broken and this was something I could not fix, nor to date can anyone fix it for me. How was I to live without myself? I wanted her back!

She was a strong and independent woman. She always tried so hard to be a loving wife, a good mother, a caring friend and a dedicated employee. She had self-confidence and enjoyed life. She never imagined that by the age of 41 she would be forced into retirement. She had not yet observed even one of her sons graduate from college, nor known the pleasures of a daughter-in-law, or held a grandchild in her arms.

Needless to say, the future did not look bright. The leader must now learn to follow. Adversities in life were once looked upon as a challenge; now they're just confusing situations that someone else must handle. Control of *my life* will slowly be relinquished to others. I must learn to trust–completely.

An intense fear enveloped my entire being as I mourned the loss of what was and the hopes and dreams that might never be. How could this be happening to me? What exactly will become of me? These questions occupied much of my time for far too many days.

Then one day as I fumbled around the kitchen to prepare a pot of coffee, something caught my eye through the window. It had snowed and I had truly forgotten what a beautiful sight a soft, gentle snowfall could be. I eagerly but so slowly dressed and went outside to join my son, who was shoveling our driveway. As I bent down to gather a mass of those radiantly white flakes on my shovel, it seemed as though I could do nothing but marvel at their beauty. Needless to say, he did not share in my enthusiasm; to him it was a job, but to me it was an experience.

Later I realized that for a short period of time, God granted me the ability to see a snowfall through the same innocent eyes of the child I once was, so many years ago. I am still here, I thought, and there will be wonders to be held in each new day; they are just different now. . . . Now my quality of life is feeding the dogs, looking at flowers. My husband says I am more content now than ever before! Love and dignity, those are the keys. This brings you back down to the basics in life, a smile makes you happy (p. 18-20)

The most remarkable theology of dementia is David Keck's (1996) *Forgetting Whose We Are: Alzheimer's Disease and the Love of God.* Keck describes the experience of his mother, who has suffered with AD for more than a decade. He asserts that aesthetic experience is still open to his mother, who seems enchanted by the beauty of a wooded path; he believes that she thrives in church, stimulated by hymns, the sense of community, and well known litanies. While her purposeful means-ends reasoning is seriously diminished, nevertheless she still seems to appreciate the glory of God's creation. Keck suggests that his mother may in some respects be closer to this appreciation of creation than the routines of our busy lives usually permit.

It is easy to be against people with dementia because our culture is against forgetfulness. We live in a culture that is the child of rationalism and capitalism, so clarity of mind and economic productivity determine the value of a human life. The dictum "I think, therefore I am," is not easily replaced with an equal appreciation for the relational, emotional, aesthetic, and spiritual aspects of well-being. We are so fearful of dementia that we draw firm diagnostic lines between "those" who are demented and "us" who are not, when in fact we are all a little demented. Post (1995) has argued that there is a tendency in a "hypercognitive culture" to exclude the deeply forgetful. An appreciation for spirituality may work against such exclusion, and this is moral gain.

People with AD as well as their caregivers can benefit remarkably from pastoral care. Sometimes, the individual who has not spoken coherently for several years will suddenly blurt out a prayer or a hymn, for such deeply learned material is the very last to disappear. The beauty of litanies, prayers, and hymns has a certain affective power. We remain open to the idea that as the capacity for technical (means to ends) rationality fades, more contemplative and spiritual capacities are elevated. Demented people continue to respond to their faith and inner needs through long-remembered rituals that connect them with the present. Prayers and hymns are still familiar in many cases, especially after several repetitions. Worship in nursing homes can create "the awareness of connectedness."

The deterioration of cognitive abilities calls out for some kind of spiritual reconstruction. Is it possible within the depths of despair for people with AD to be spiritually enriched? Indeed, this may be worthy of much fuller study, but the emergence of spirituality in AD has not yet been examined. Quality of life assessment in dementia is in a rudimentary stage, but becoming increasingly important in the evaluation of new treatments and health care interventions. How can one assess quality of life when an individual has communication and memory problems that preclude response. Yet there is the possibility that assessment measures will become refined even in such cases, allowing the impact of spiritual and religious practice to be understood more clearly.

THE PLACE OF PRAYER IN THE LIVES OF CAREGIVERS

Caregivers often pray for loved ones with dementia. According to most rabbinic opinion, the claim that God must answer a prayer is presumptuous and represents a transgression. In the words of Reissner, the Hebrew Bible and the Talmud indicate that prayer is thought to be efficacious if offered by the proper person at the proper time with the proper intent and under the proper circumstances (Reissner 1986).

The fact remains that the vast majority of humankind prays for the sick. This is clearly the case with family members caring for loved ones with AD. In a recent study of religiosity variables in relation to perceived caregiver rewards, African-American women caring for elderly persons with major deficits in activities of daily living perceived benefits through caring based on a spiritual-religious reframing of their situation. Religiosity indicators (i.e., "prayer, comfort from religion, self-rated religiosity, attendance at religious services") are especially significant as coping resources in African-American women caregivers (Picot et al. 1997). Religiosity is a clear stress deterrent, and therefore also impacts depression rates, which are extraordinarily high in AD caregivers. These authors suggest that "if religiosity indicators are shown to enhance a caregiver's perceived rewards, health care professionals could encourage caregivers to use their religiosity to reduce the negative consequences and increase the rewards of caregiving" (Picot et al., p. 89). This seems self-evident.

From a purely economic perspective, the spirituality of caregivers can sustain their abilities to care, and thus keep people with AD out of nursing homes longer. While this is an ambiguous goal, the fact is that nursing home care costs families and the medicaid system a great deal of money.

CONCLUSIONS

AD raises the post modernist question of the dominance of rationality in our conception of the human self. The slow disintegration of components of thought and eventually, feeling, found in AD raises the basic question: what does it mean to be human?

The concept of spirituality is broad, encompassing many human behaviors and beliefs. Nevertheless, we believe that clues to understanding spiritual practices and beliefs can be found through brain studies. Perhaps some of the most interesting observations have been made in the spiritual events that occur in the course of schizophrenia and temporal lobe epilepsy. Some temporal lobe epileptics develop a profound sense of spirituality (hyper religiosity). It is possible to ask whether states in which the brain is damaged in more obvious ways such as dementia can help us understand the neurological substrates of spirituality.

Thus the relationships between AD and spirituality are many and deserve further exploration. If invoked and supported, spirituality can enhance the quality of life of all those involved. Additionally, an exploration of spirituality in those with AD can enrich our understanding of the neurological and psychological aspects of hope, prayer, and the power of belief. We look forward to a better empirical understanding of how chaplains can best serve the spiritual needs and capacities of those vulnerable among us with AD.

REFERENCES

Anderson J.M., Anderson L.J., and Felsenthal G. 1993. Pastoral Needs for Support Within an Inpatient Rehabilitation Unit. *Archives of Physical Medicine and Rehabilitation* 74,574-578.

Davis R. (with help from his wife Betty). (1989). *My Journey into Alzheimer's Disease: Helpful Insights for Family and Friends.* Wheaton, Il.: Tyndale House.

Everett D. 1997. "Forget Me Not: The Spiritual Care of People with Alzheimer's," *Proceedings of the Sixth National Alzheimer's Disease Education Conference.* Chicago: Alzheimer's Association, July 20-23, 1997, A4.

Frankl V. 1963. *Man's Search for Meaning.* Boston: Beacon Press.

Keck D. 1996. *Forgetting Whose We Are: Alzheimer's Disease and the Love of God.* Nashville: Abington.

Khalsa D.S. 1996. New Developments in the Prevention and Reversal of Memory Loss. In: *Advances in Anti-Aging Medicine,* R.M.Klatz, ed. New York: Mary Ann Liebert, pp. 13-17.

Larson D.B., and Milano M.A. 1995. Are Religion and Spirituality Clinically Relevant in Health Care? *Mind/Body Medicine* 1, 147-157.

Lupien S., Lecours A., and Lussier I. 1994. Basan Cortisol Levels and Cognitive Deficits in Human Aging. *Journal of Neuroscience* 14, 2893-2903.

Maugans T.A. 1996. The SPIRITual history. *Archives of Family Medicine* 5, 11-16.

Picot S.J., Debanne, S.M., Namazi K.H., Wykle M.L. 1997. Religiosity and Perceived Rewards of Black and White Caregivers. *The Gerontologist* 37(1), 89-101.

Post S.G. 1995. *The Moral Challenge of Alzheimer Disease.* Baltimore, Md.: Johns Hopkins University Press.

Reissner F. 1986. *Modern Medicine and Jewish Ethics.* New York: Yeshiva University Press, 1986.

Sacks O. 1970. The Lost Mariner. In: *The Man Who Mistook His Wife for a Hat and Other Clinical Tales.* New York: HarperCollins, pp. 23-42.

Sapolsky R. 1992. *Stress: The Aging Brain and the Mechanism of Neuron Death.* Cambridge, Ma.: MIT Press.

Underwood-Gordon L. 1995. *A Working Model of Health: Spirituality and Religiousness as Resources: Applications to Persons with Disability.* National Institutes of Health.

Pastoral Care
of Problematic Alzheimer's Disease
and Dementia Affected Residents
in a Long-Term Care Setting

David P. Wentroble, MDiv, BCC

SUMMARY. Pastoral caregivers face many challenges in providing ministry to institutional persons with dementia. This article describes the psychosocial perspective of Bowlby concerning the management of persons with dementia and a pastoral care ministry based on it. Specific pastoral programs and interventions are described. The article contains four case studies and concludes with reflections concerning the chaplain's ministry. *[Article copies available for a fee from The Haworth Document Delivery Service: 1-800-342-9678. E-mail address: getinfo@haworthpressinc.com]*

On November 5, 1994 Alzheimer's Disease (AD) received a great boost of recognition! Former President Ronald Reagan released a letter to the American public announcing that he was afflicted with the disease. In that moment, AD acquired a human face. Suddenly all of America confronted a disease that affects thousands of persons and families and church members. A disease often seen from a distance on television, or read about dispassionately from a newsweekly now touched the hearts of millions.

David P. Wentroble is affiliated with the Greenwich Chaplaincy Services, Greenwich, CT.

[Haworth co-indexing entry note]: "Pastoral Care of Problematic Alzheimer's Disease and Dementia Affected Residents in a Long-Term Care Setting." Wentroble, David P. Co-published simultaneously in *Journal of Health Care Chaplaincy* (The Haworth Pastoral Press, an imprint of The Haworth Press, Inc.) Vol. 8, No. 1/2, 1999, pp. 59-76; and: *Spiritual Care for Persons with Dementia: Fundamentals for Pastoral Practice* (ed: Larry VandeCreek) The Haworth Pastoral Press, an imprint of The Haworth Press, Inc., 1999, pp. 59-76. Single or multiple copies of this article are available for a fee from The Haworth Document Delivery Service [1-800-342-9678, 9:00 a.m. - 5:00 p.m. (EST). E-mail address: getinfo@haworthpressinc.com].

The increased level of primary medical care creates a much older population. Once people lived for only a few years after retirement; now there are active and healthy 70, 80 and even 90 year-olds, and the number of people over the century mark is increasing. One of the unfortunate side-effects of all this progress is the increase of diseases rarely seen before. Since people are living longer, diseases such as AD have more opportunity to strike.

The Merck Manual of Geriatrics (Abrams, Beers, and Berkow 1995, p. 1148) defines AD as a "progressive neuropsychiatric disease, found sometimes in middle-aged and more often in older adults, that affects brain matter and is characterized by the inexorable loss of cognitive function as well as by affective and behavioral disturbances."

AD's primary effect is on the cognitive function of the individual. While there are many physiological affects, the resident with AD primarily exhibits behaviors of dementia which lead to the problems of proper caregiving.

Alan Siegel, M.D. (1994) of the Alzheimer's Resource Center of Connecticut notes that, while in 1994 there were 4 million Americans with an AD diagnosis, by the year 2040, there will be in excess of 8 million cases in people over age 65. At the time of his report, 50% of nursing home residents had a primary or secondary diagnosis of AD. Data reported by L.E. Hebert (1995) support this data.

While general physical care, food, shelter, clothing and the activities of daily living are generally well taken care of, the pastoral realm of life for those with AD is woefully neglected. This neglect is more out of a sense of helplessness than an unwillingness to help, but to work with people with AD is often to work seemingly with no goal in sight, no new horizon to conquer, no progress to be made.

In *Activities with Persons Disabled by Alzheimer's Disease and Related Disorders* [ADRD], Carol Bowlby (1993, p. 39-40) outlines the stages of Alzheimer's Disease:

> In the early stages of AD the changes are so subtle that neither the individual nor significant others may take particular note of the changes. The hallmark symptom of AD, memory loss, appears at this stage. This memory loss is periodic and inconsistent and occurs particularly in unfamiliar surroundings. . . . The individual becomes less and less able to cope in unfamiliar settings and experiences frequent disorientation as to place and time.

Difficulties with communication, written and verbal, become more apparent. . . . Motor coordination problems appear, and are more pronounced for some than for others. . . . Frustration with the progressive losses may lead to extreme emotional reactions, or catastrophic reactions, to seemingly minor events. . . . Cognitive function is greatly impaired, and the learning of new material, especially verbal material, is very difficult. . . . In the advanced stage, verbal cues usually are not sufficient, and the individual requires constant supervision and physical assistance for personal activities such as toileting and personal hygiene. . . . In the terminal stage, the Alzheimer's patient is totally dependent on others. The patient may be unable to move, speak, or swallow. . . . The complications of AD in this stage lead to death.

Since so much of the behavior of the Alzheimer's affected resident can be problematic, including wandering, disruptive verbalizations, stressful encounters with peers that can lead to physical attacks, the pastoral caregiver must determine how to best minister to them while not neglecting their real needs.

There are many barriers to cross. How can we understand what the AD patient is trying to express to us? For the AD patient, things are being expressed that make sense to themselves, yet they cannot communicate properly to others. Joseph Foley (1992, p. 40) writes, "The very nature of dementia makes it difficult and in some cases impossible to learn what thought processes and what feelings lie behind the distorted behaviors."

To begin mapping out the structure of pastoral care to the resident with AD, we need to look at what behaviors, what parts of a person's memory, and what functions persist in the resident. Bowlby (1993, p. 45) points out that there are many behaviors that are very ingrained in people, such as shaking hands and smiling. By simply reaching out a hand and saying "Hello," many people who are debilitated are able to respond with a smile, an outstretched hand or their own "Hello."

Touch is an important facilitator in achieving a sense of worth, that someone is indeed caring for "me" and is an important start to group interactions. Bowlby (1993, p. 45) again: "By supporting and encouraging sociability in groups and with individuals, this persisting skill can help to compensate for losses in memory, reasoning, and language."

Bowlby (1993, p. 43-44) writes of the "persisting assets" that remain with those with AD and need to be recognized and utilized in their care: "emotional awareness and emotional memory; sensory appreciation; primary motor function; sociability and social skills; procedural memory/habitual skills; long-term memory; sense of humor."

Jitka M. Zgola (1987, p. 21) writes in a similar vein, "Programs should take maximal advantage of the ability to perform overlearned or habitual tasks, primary motor and sensory functions, emotional awareness, remote memory, and the tendency to perseverate."

While some might argue that these people should just be cared for in their basic human needs–food, clothing, bathing, help in toileting– there is really a need for more supportive activities, things to tap into those persisting assets, and help the overall life of the ADRD individual and also lead to appropriate pastoral care for the individual. Bowlby (1993, p. 55) points out that if the special care needs of the AD patient are neglected, the course of the disease leads into a downward spiral in all sorts of functions, not simply physical ones. The person's mentation, thinking processes, problem solving skills, and communication skills all decline and any attempt at independence is likely to have little success. It is therefore quite important that we utilize all the resources that the resident has available to enrich their life as much as possible.

In approaching the area of spiritual activities, Bowlby (1993, p. 164) cites research pointing out the central importance of religious activities to those with AD. "Religious behavior was the most frequently reported coping behavior. Forty-five percent of the sample reported religious behavior as a way of coping with one of the three stressful life events described. Seventy-five percent of these religious coping behaviors were related to personal religious attitudes, such as faith, trust in God, and private prayer."

At The Nathaniel Witherell, a municipal nursing home in Greenwich, Connecticut, the residents come from many faith groups, primarily Roman Catholic, Episcopalian, and Congregational. One must realize that in working with such a diverse group, one has to be sensitive to differences and similarities. Bowlby (1993, p. 164) writes,

Supporting the person with ADRD in maintaining lifelong religious practices requires great sensitivity to both the disease process and to personal beliefs. The activity specialist's role is interpreting the disease processes and working with a religious leader, volunteer, or family member of the same faith, in order to adapt religious activities to the individual's present abilities. . . . Inclusion in religious activities must be based on lifelong practices, and care must be taken not to offend family members and significant others.

Spiritual and pastoral care together help the person hold onto the important aspects of his or her faith. Retaining connection to people, words and Word, rites, rituals, music, pictures and the like will all help the ADRD resident keep a base of spirituality from which to draw inner strength.

At the time the need was recognized for such special pastoral care, I served as chaplain at three nursing homes in Greenwich, Connecticut, serving through the auspices of Greenwich Chaplaincy Services, an interfaith organization. In 1993, Greenwich Woods Health Care Center, one of the three homes, opened a new wing specifically designed for persons with AD and related dementias [ADRD]. Later, The Nathaniel Witherell, a skilled nursing facility, through the reassigning of rooms, shifted residents around to create an enhanced recreation unit specifically for persons with AD. At that time I provided worship and Bible-study opportunities at these homes for most of the residents. Now, however, the AD units were segregating out a good percentage of the population. These people were kept on their units for more attention and better and more specific care. Because persons with AD have very special needs, being in a separate unit allowed them to be given better care. Such a move also made patient care easier for the staff. An unfortunate side-effect was that these residents were excluded from the worship and pastoral care life of the homes. When they would take part in group activities elsewhere, e.g., the regular chapel service, very often they would be disruptive, and this was quite disturbing to the more alert residents. The administration and staffs of the homes were aware of the need for increased pastoral care and worship opportunities for these residents and asked me to provide such services. This pastoral care had to be carefully crafted so as to recognize the special care concerns of the residents with AD. Services that worked in other units could not simply be transferred to these units, but special forms of worship and pastoral care had to be developed. These forms needed to include a great deal of visual, aural and vocal stimulation, things to keep people's attention. Activities needed to be available to stimulate the senses: smell, taste, touch, sight, hearing.

The primary focus was small group worship experiences enhanced with the use of religious objects in reminiscence packets. Bowlby (1993, p. 45) points out, "Groups are a particularly good setting for encouraging social skills."

Bowlby (1993, p. 97) discusses working with groups of Alzheimer's patients in general and religious activities in particular in her book. In working with such patients we must recognize that those with dementia have as great a need for group structure as other people. The style of such groups must compensate for weaknesses and accentuate the strengths of the participants. With such adjustments taken into account, the person with dementia may actually experience a great deal of positive involvement, personal growth, and a positive contribution to the total group. When working with groups, Bowlby (1993, p. 97-98) says we must recognize that:

- Groups fill a basic human need for belonging and togetherness. . . .
- Groups are a natural, normal, and adult setting for socialization and activities that make use of the persisting asset of sociability. . . .
- The social atmosphere of a group encourages social behavior, participation, and normal adult function . . .
- The more disabled members of the group pattern their behavior on that of more highly functioning members. . . .
- Group members, enabled by staff, provide support and encouragement for each other.

As far as the type of activities to use, Bowlby (1993, p. 105-106) suggests to recall overlearned, very familiar activities, such as shaking hands, playing catch, . . . are simple, repetitive, but ADULT activities, . . . emphasize the ability to appreciate sensory experiences, such as feeling a fur muff or a felt hat; . . . emphasize overlearned and persistent social skills, such as greeting one another, . . . emphasize the ability to participate in gross motor activities, such as dancing, moving to music, . . . emphasize remote memory, especially childhood and young-adult memories, and provide an opportunity for reminiscence; . . . provide an opportunity for active participation, such as . . . singing, humming, or clapping with music. . . . have an obvious or identifiable purpose, . . . emphasize nonverbal skills, such as responding to music, . . . provide immediate positive feedback, . . .

As far as the actual activity is concerned, Bowlby (1993, p. 106-107) writes,

> Use ample familiar, concrete physical cues and memorabilia. . . . Use multisensory cues. . . . Include one or two participants who are high functioning and will respond well to the group. These individuals serve as a model and as a stimulus for others to participate. . . . Make an agenda and a written plan. . . . Plan to take the initiative throughout the group, as most persons with ADRD are unable to do so for themselves. Always be ready to adapt. . . . Do not expect to be able to run a traditional group, with everyone following the group leader and doing the same thing at the same time. . . . Provide a bridge from the general milieu of the day room or unit to the group and back again. . . .

In evaluating the group, here are some questions to be asked (Bowlby 1993, p. 109):

- Does the person appear calm and happy in the group?
- After a period of involvement, does the person appear pleased when seeing you and/or the group setting?
- Does the person respond verbally and/or nonverbally?
- How long does the activity hold attention? Does the activity create social exchange between participants?
- Do the participants appear content? Do the participants become restless?
- Is it difficult to return participants to the general milieu?

Music is a very important component of working with ADRD residents. "In neurological terms, the 'musical' areas of the brain are usually in the nondominant hemisphere, the side of the brain that does not control language. Appreciating, responding to, and becoming involved in music do not require the areas of the brain that are usually damaged by the disease processes of ADRD. . . . In one study, the use of music during a reminiscence group resulted in higher measures of life satisfaction and a greater level of enjoyment, compared to a control group which did not use music" (Bowlby, 1993, p. 155).

As to the reasons for having religious activities with those affected with AD, Bowlby (1993, p. 165) lists the following:

- They are a recognized source of support and reassurance during the stress of coping with ADRD.
- They provide an opportunity for spiritual and emotional expression.
- They are familiar and reassuring activities that call upon over-learned, familiar activities and behaviors.
- They are an important part of the life experience of many; thus they are essential to holistic treatment.
- They represent a unique way of communicating, which can be very meaningful when standard communication fails.
- They are meaningful, adult activities. They provide an opportunity for reminiscence.

In following such a model, the group in a nursing home setting becomes a real community of faith. As nursing homes and other facilities gear up for an ever-increasing case load of Alzheimer's patients, the area of religious activities has been recognized as essential. The above group guidelines give a bit of direction and structure and indeed have a "spiritual" sense about them. In discussing the use of religious activities, Bowlby (1993, p. 165) gives some thoughts about being sensitive to the broad diversity of religious faiths present. The caregiver must be aware of the religious backgrounds of the residents. They must plan pastoral care in consultation with a religious leader from the respective groups. Special religious activities should be planned around religious festivals and holidays using music, symbols and other items that may elicit religious responses. While we often work in a group setting, we must not forget the importance of one-on-one pastoral encounters.

As far as the concerns of loss of memory, Elaine Ramshaw (1987, p. 81) writes "The familiarity of ritual may offset even severe impairments of memory. I have heard again and again from pastors that ritual order will trigger a familiar, lifelong memory pattern even in senile people who are not tracking at all well in the present."

With regard to the importance of liturgical memory, she (1987, p. 93) writes,

The source of liturgy's power to challenge is in its memory. Liturgical remembrance is a unique sort of memory: a memory which does not just reminisce but re-presents, makes present; a memory which by recalling the promises of the past also recalls our future hope. The paradigmatic act of liturgical memory is the anamnesis of the eucharistic prayer, where the historical acts and future promises of God are recalled and re-presented in the act and promise of God's Christ in our midst, the covenant of bread and wine. Here we recall the history of Israel, of Jesus, and of the church as the history of God's self-giving. In this recollection we know who we are in the present: the outcome of God's creative love, the children of God adopted in baptism, the younger siblings of the Jews in the history of covenant, the followers of Jesus in the way of the cross. In this same recollection we also remember the promises God has made about our future, when Christ will come again and the reign of God will begin.

In an article in the *Journal of Pastoral Care*, Chaplain Jean Clayton (1991, p. 178) affirms the use of such resources:

Since the "message" is meant to be largely interpretative or instructional, the logical functions of the left-brain are called into action–functions no longer easily accessed by many elders, particularly the memory impaired. Yet, familiar scripture, music, prayers, and symbols retain their power to touch many of the same people through the feeling functions of the right brain. This approach matched that of many Alzheimer's caregivers who used music, aroma, touch, and other emotionally powerful ways of "reaching" patients long after all memory had failed.

Likewise, Lisa Gwyther (1995) points out that for those with religious backgrounds, certain symbols of faith elicit responses. Rather than having to think cognitively, one's emotions become more apparent. The appearance of a cross, a Star of David, a clerical collar, vestments elicit great emotions. Touching a Bible, a prayer-book or a rosary can also spark emotions that will make connections to religious activities of the past.

Another author, Thomas St. James O'Connor (1992, p. 11) also utilizes many religious objects:

I thought of traditional religious symbols that could be helpful. As the head nurse reminded me, these people grew up in the early part of this century and would recognize a man in a collar as a pastoral care worker rather than a man in a suit with a name tag. I decided to use some traditional religious symbols that patients could see, touch, hear, and smell. I used: A Roman collar; A Bible; Holy cards with Bible scenes; Hymns on a tape recorder; A stuffed lamb; Traditional prayers.

At The Nathaniel Witherell, the times of pastoral care become rather joyous and loud. Since AD residents can become disruptive, we thought it best to have two people present so that one could continue the program while the other could spend time with a disruptive resident, if necessary. As it turns out, nearly every time we meet a need occurs that calls one of us to deal with the special needs of an individual. I am very blessed to have Suzanne Testani, a Therapeutic Recreation Director, assist me with the group.

We hold the group meeting twice a week for about a half-hour each. Depending on the day and the alertness level of the residents, we have anywhere from ten to twenty residents participating. Of that number, perhaps only half are able to respond, yet it is my sense that the others who are in the room benefit from the group also. On those days when only one person is available to lead the group, I find that ten is about the limit for good interaction.

The group begins with our introducing ourselves and explaining that we are here to have a time of singing and prayer and story, a sort of church time. Indeed, as soon as I enter the room with the ball and my bag of stuffed lambs and robe, many residents seem to know what is soon to begin. As I robe, I explain the various pieces and point out the colors and shapes on the stoles.

The sessions starts out with a ball-toss of an inflated world globe, while singing "He's Got the Whole World in His Hands," a song familiar to most of the residents. The tossing of the ball is a very good activity for those with AD and provides a focus for the beginning of the pastoral care time. Some residents are able to catch the ball and throw it back while others have some difficulty. For the latter we touch their hands with the ball, making sure that all residents have a chance to participate. I then often ask, "Who is the 'He' that we are singing about?" and very often I get a "The Lord" from one to a few residents. The time then progresses with a few more familiar songs, e.g., "Jesus Loves Me," "Jesus Loves the Little Children," and Christmas carols during the Advent/Christmas season. We then pass out the stuffed sheep, asking the resident to help us by holding onto the sheep. I then read the 23rd Psalm, introducing it as "something you probably have heard before." I pause at strategic places to hear if anyone is speaking along, and quite often I hear some of the residents say "Shepherd," after I say "The Lord is my. . . . " "And I shall dwell in the house of the Lord. . . . " gets many people to say "Forever. Amen." I then ask the group if anyone knows that, and if so, what is it? Some will say "A prayer"; others "a Psalm"; and some, such as Luke and Gloria, will say "The 23rd Psalm."

I explain that the sheep are reminders to us that God loves us, as a shepherd loves his sheep. While that might be difficult for many to understand, I have found in the course of the pastoral care group that the sheep now stand for God's love for several of the residents (see the vignette concerning Luke below). I give a very brief "meditation" utilizing an object or picture, perhaps talking about God as our "Rock" and asking people what a rock is like and if God is at all like that. I often lead an antiphonal Psalm, the 150th, asking the residents to echo me, and they do it surprisingly well.

During the entire time, both the recreation therapist and I circulate through the room, taking hands and moving people's arms along with the rhythm of the music. We begin to come to a close by asking the group if they know what prayer is, and Gloria or Luke respond with "Talking to God," "Time with the Lord," or something similar. When I ask what is the most familiar prayer, one of the residents often says "The Lord's Prayer." It is interesting that someone will often say "The 23rd Psalm," and I will acknowledge that that too is a prayer, and there is an even more familiar one. I will usually ask the person who first said "The Lord's Prayer" if they can start it for the group, and they often will, "Our Father. . . . " The time closes with the singing of *Amazing Grace* and a benediction during which many people cross themselves. Suzanne and I then greet each resident individually with a handshake, an important tactile time for them and for us, and we remind everyone that we will be back in a few days to do the group again.

From time to time I have a service of communion, explaining what the bread and wine mean. I know from my experience and reading that the tactile nature of communion is so very important to so many, especially to those who cannot respond in any way. The responses of the residents vary from time to time. Some residents readily accept the wafer, while others have no idea what to do with it. One man always removes his ever-present hat whenever I serve him the elements.

An important second aspect to the pastoral care was the utilization of reminiscence packets. These were packets of significant religious objects. Such objects include prayer cards, rosaries, crosses, Bibles and other objects that might elicit memories. The use of tactile objects seems to be helpful in bringing back memories. The packets are provided for family members to use with their resident. We prepared three different packets, one for Roman Catholics, one for Protestants, and one for Jewish residents.

In the Catholic one we included the following:

- Crucifix
- Rosary and How to Say the Rosary
- Scapular
- Sacred Heart Badge
- Statue of Mary
- Common Catholic Prayers
- Prayer Cards:
  - The Lord's Prayer
  - 23rd Psalm
  - The Ten Commandments
  - Apostles' Creed
  - The Hail Mary
  - Magnificat
  - Mysteries of the Holy Rosary
  - Prayer to the Sacred Heart

The Protestant Packet included:

- Bible *(New King James Version)*
- Cross
- *A Companion of Prayer for Daily Living*
- Traditional Picture of Jesus
- Scripture and Prayer Cards:
  - The Lord's Prayer
  - 23rd Psalm
  - The Ten Commandments
  - Numbers 6:24-26

The Jewish Packet included:

- Prayer Book
- Yarmulkes (2)
- Prayer Shawls (2)
- Tefillin
- Mezuzah
- Candlesticks

These packets were assembled in consultation with local clergy. They have been well used by family members.

In addition to the groups and family use of the reminiscence packets, one-on-one encounters are very important. These consist of encounters one to three times a week with each resident. Time is spent in talking, in prayer, often using the Lord's Prayer, in Bible reading, usually using familiar passages such as the 23rd Psalm. We also spend time utilizing the religious objects found in the various reminiscence packets. In addition, whenever I am on the unit, as I encounter the individual resident, I will hold their hands and start out the Lord's Prayer or the 23rd Psalm. I do this more with those residents unable to come to the group, because it is very important to let the resident know that there is still a connection to their faith community even in the surroundings of a nursing home.

Ideally, all three parts, worship group, reminiscence packets, and one-on-ones are used with the majority of the residents. Certain ones respond better in the one-on-one encounter or with family than with the group. Suzanne and I recognize that each resident, though affected by the same disease, remain individuals, each with a unique need for pastoral support.

VIGNETTES

The most vivid way to show the validity of the special pastoral care is through the use of vignettes, brief narratives of some of the responses of the residents. The names have been changed.

Stella

Stella is a very frustrating subject on the unit. From the beginning of the special pastoral care group to the present time, she has not changed. She is always antagonistic, vowing to "call the police!" or offering some other such threat. While she can be quite charming to her son, to anyone else, including staff and other residents, she is cantankerous.

She always has a stuffed animal of some sort with her, and when we started using the stuffed sheep she began to claim that they were hers. We found out the hard way not to let her hold one of our sheep, for she would not give it up at the end of the group time.

She is present at every pastoral care group event, so I hope that perhaps some of the music, the words of Scripture or prayers may be touching her in some way. An interesting side note is that Stella once played the piano. Whenever her son visits, they sit together at the piano and she tries to play along with him, with a modicum of success at times!

Stella's lack of response to the pastoral care appears to be due to the advanced stage of her dementia. This raises the important question of how to give even more appropriate pastoral care to those at similar levels to Stella.

Luke

Luke has shown the greatest response to the pastoral care group. He came to The Nathaniel Witherell with a long history of Episcopal Church background, having been a choirboy years ago and remaining active in the church into his adult life. When we started the group, he would easily blow-up at inconsequential events. As we progressed, he began to sing more, to recognize scripture passages such as the 23rd Psalm, and was soon able to lead the group in the Lord's Prayer.

As he participated more, more surprising things occurred. One day we were singing "This Little Light of Mine," and I asked the group, "Where should we let our lights shine?" Nothing was forthcoming from anybody, so I suggested Greenwich, to which Luke replied, "The whole world needs it, not just Greenwich!" Even in the midst of his dementia, Luke was able to grasp the concept of the song, that God calls us to "shine" our faith everywhere. For Luke, the Town of Greenwich was too limited a place to shine his faith. He realized that he needed to shine it throughout the world. A brief deep bit of insight and a moment of serendipity!

Luke's wife is a frequent visitor, and often takes part in the pastoral care group meetings. During the recent Christmas season, as we were singing carols, I asked the group, "What carols could we sing that referred to snow?" since it was, at that point, snowing outside. Hearing no response, I suggested "Good King Wenceslas," and we started singing. In general, I know the first verse of most carols, but I was stymied after " . . . deep and crisp and even." To the surprise of Luke's wife, me and the other staff present, Luke continued with the correct words, "Brightly shone the moon that night, Though the frost was cruel, When a poor man came in sight, Gath'ring winter fuel."

Luke's response to the pastoral care group has been phenomenal. He is the most active and vocal participant, and as shown above, often adds more than expected to the group. Luke is always glad to be holding one of the stuffed lambs, and when I ask the group if they know why I bring the sheep, Luke often says, "They show us that God loves us." Lately though, Luke has also become fond of flinging his lamb in the midst of the worship group. He always makes sure that one of us is watching as he does the deed!

As his disease has progressed, Luke often gets more emotional, often crying during some of the music. One of us usually goes to be by his side at such times to offer some comforting words or touch.

Gloria

Gloria is a surprising latecomer to the group. She had been a wanderer, and it was difficult to keep her attention. After some falls and a lot of unsteadiness, it was decided to confine her to a special chair on wheels, one more protective of her than a normal wheelchair. She was still able to wander, but now she had the support and safety of the chair. She would sometimes wander into the room where we were having the group meeting, and then shortly thereafter wander out. After some time, though, she began to stay and to join in on some of the songs. After a while, she was able to lead the group in the Lord's Prayer and the 23rd Psalm, and is now as alert and responsive as Luke.

It seems to the nursing staff that Gloria's good response is much due to her being in a special chair that still gives her freedom, but offers a great deal of protection from falls. It seems that she is better able to concentrate on the activities of the group when she does not have to worry about her balance. She also has the freedom to leave the group, and on some occasions she still does, but often returns to the group towards the end of the session.

Letty

Letty is a special blessing to the group, for in addition to her AD diagnosis, she has Down's Syndrome. Often prone to crying fits for no apparent reason, Letty is present most days in the group, but has to be taken out if she gets to be too disruptive for the others. Some days she is fine, smiling at me and Suzanne as we approach her, but not really showing any response to the activity.

We discovered that Letty knew the song "Kum Ba Yah" and that it was her favorite song. From then on, before we would sing it, I or one of the other helpers would go to Letty and ask her, "Letty, what is your favorite song?" Quite often she would reply, "Kum Ba Yah," and together we would start singing it.

Unfortunately, Letty's condition has declined recently. She still attends the group, she still looks up at me or the others leading, but she will not sing "Kum Ba Yah" any more. We are sure to sing it for her, and the group, and remind them that it is Letty's favorite song. Because we know that, and the group knows that, Letty is really able to participate and is an important and valuable member of the group.

Letty is also one of those who we want to keep in the group, even though she is unable to respond. She had been an important part of the group when it began and she continues to be essential, even though she no longer responds. Some of the other residents also appear to enjoy her presence often by offering her their stuffed lambs.

Letty's decline points out the importance a single individual has for the group. She is an essential member of the group even if she cannot contribute. The other residents recognize her presence, and I think that they would miss her if she was no longer present in the group.

Reflections

As I reflect on this past work with the Alzheimer's residents and look to the future with them, I am overcome with the many images of the residents, fingering rosaries and saying "Hail Mary. . . ." I remember their learning of new songs and remembering of old ones. I hear the echoes of the Antiphonal Psalm 150, the gentle words of the 23rd Psalm, the familiar cadence of The Lord's Prayer, and I realize that I have been greatly rewarded.

Two strong lessons came through this work. First, there needs to be more education about nursing homes in general, and AD in particular to the general public. When I began this work in 1993 I looked for some volunteers from local churches. I was astonished at the lack of response to my request. While The Nathaniel Witherell Auxiliary has a large number of volunteers who come in each week to serve the residents, none was willing to work with the AD residents. When I contacted the local clergy, explained the program and requested volunteers, there was only one respondent from the members of the churches, and that person was inappropriate for the project.

While I realize that each person has a different gift for ministry, this lack of response shows me that at the very least I need to do more education in the local congregations. In talking with both clergy and present volunteers, it appears that the reticence in volunteering is due to a fear of not knowing how to interact with someone with dementia. Most people want to be able to converse intelligently with someone. There is no problem at The Nathaniel Witherell getting volunteers willing to talk with totally bed-bound people who are able to talk intelligently and interact with others.

I have met with several adult study groups at local churches, and those attending confirmed my suspicions. Some admitted a bit of anxiety over "what to do" when visiting someone with AD. As I explained the course of the disease and some possibilities for interaction, for example, utilizing the various reminiscence packets, a few people expressed a willingness to think about giving it a try. More churches are inviting me in to speak or preach about this ministry, and the responses have been heartening.

The second strong lesson is to perpetually remember that each resident is an individual with his or her own special needs. I realize that this seems to be too obvious of a statement, yet so often in nursing home care we generalize. "Oh, that's an AD resident. We'll just do thus and so for their care." "Mr. Smith had a stroke, so we'll care for him in this way." In a nursing home setting, persons have the possibility of becoming so dehumanized, turned into a number, an object, a statistic, a bed in a room. From the time of their admission to the time of their death, each resident deserves to be treated as a separate individual, one of God's flock to be loved, cared for, paid attention to.

In the course of this program I worked with people ranging in response from Stella to Luke and many people in between. Each encounter was an adventure, there was no guarantee that today's group was going to behave like last Tuesday's. Each one-on-one was different as people said the Lord's Prayer, the 23rd Psalm, or the rosary, and touched the various objects that contained such very deep spiritual meanings.

During the course of this work, I was in the presence of the Spirit of God every time I encountered one of the AD residents. In that interaction, whether brief or long, I received much more from the resident than I gave to them. The Spirit of God is so very present and active and alive in these ADRD residents, in the "least of these" our sisters and brothers.

REFERENCES

Abrams, W. B., Beers, M.H., Berkow, R. (eds). 1995. *The Merck manual of geriatrics* (2nd edition), Whitehour Station, NJ: Merck and Co., Inc.

Bowlby, C. 1993. *Therapeutic activities with persons disabled by Alzheimer's disease and related disorders.* Gaithersburg: Aspen Publishers.

Clayton, J. 1991. Let there be life: An approach to worship with Alzheimer's patients and their families. *The Journal of Pastoral Care* 45 (Summer).

Foley, J. 1992. The experience of being demented. In: Robert Binstock, Stephen Post, and Peter Whitehours (eds). *Dementia and aging.* Baltimore: The Johns Hopkins University Press.

Gwyther L. 1995. *You are one of us.* Durham: Duke University Medical Center.

Hebert L.E. 1995. Age-specific incidence of Alzheimer's disease in a community population. *JAMA* 273 (May 3), 1354-1359.

Ramshaw, E. 1987. *Ritual and pastoral care.* Philadelphia: Fortress Press.

Siegel, A. 1994. *Rebuilding communication in Alzheimer's disease.* Alzheimer's Resource Center of Connecticut, March 15.

St. James O'Connor, T. 1992, Spring. Ministry without a future: A pastoral care approach to patients with senile dementia. *The Journal of Pastoral Care* 46.

Zgola, J. 1987. *Doing things.* Baltimore: The Johns Hopkins University Press.

Forget Me Not:
The Spiritual Care
of People with Alzheimer's Disease

Debbie Everett, MDiv

SUMMARY. This article observes that many clergy do not seem to understand the importance of ministry to persons with dementia. New understandings about the relationship between dementia and spirituality are presented and theological foundations explored. The article ends with a discussion of pastoral strategies that are important in this ministry. *[Article copies available for a fee from The Haworth Document Delivery Service: 1-800-342-9678. E-mail address: getinfo@haworthpressinc.com]*

Providing for the spiritual care for people with dementia has become a fairly new focus in health care. Caregivers and families of those affected are certainly interested. They are looking for support and understanding in their difficult situations.

In the eight years that I have been involved in pastoral care, it has become clear that some settings are more popular for chaplains than others. Pediatrics as well as emergency and palliative care are attractive. In these areas, chaplains are often thrown into adrenalin precipitating crises and the care of those in the "prime" of life. Certainly these are important areas of ministry that need well prepared caregivers.

Chaplain Debbie Everett is affiliated with The General Hospital of Edmonton, Edmonton, Alberta, Canada.

[Haworth co-indexing entry note]: "Forget Me Not: The Spiritual Care of People with Alzheimer's Disease." Everett, Debbie. Co-published simultaneously in *Journal of Health Care Chaplaincy* (The Haworth Pastoral Press, an imprint of The Haworth Press, Inc.) Vol. 8, No. 1/2, 1999, pp. 77-88; and: *Spiritual Care for Persons with Dementia: Fundamentals for Pastoral Practice* (ed: Larry VandeCreek) The Haworth Pastoral Press, an imprint of The Haworth Press, Inc., 1999, pp. 77-88. Single or multiple copies of this article are available for a fee from The Haworth Document Delivery Service [1-800-342-9678, 9:00 a.m. - 5:00 p.m. (EST). E-mail address: getinfo@haworthpressinc.com].

My aim in this article, however, is to offer reasons why it is difficult to find chaplains who look at long term care with the frail elderly as a place of ministry that holds as much fulfillment and meaning. My second aim is to suggest how this demanding ministry can be approached in creative ways.

The importance of this ministry needs to be addressed not only for chaplains, but also for many parish clergy who may provide pastoral care to those in their faith community affected by dementia. I have noted an ongoing struggle with some of them as to how to manage this ministry. Some ministers do not even realize the problems involved. The following example illustrates this.

One day a community clergy person inquired as to the topic of my masters thesis. I stated it was the spiritual care of people suffering from dementia. This minister paused for a moment, looked at me with a quizzical stare and then said, "why?"

This response stunned me for a moment because I found much fulfillment in this area of ministry. It offers much opportunity for the expression of the love of God to both residents and family members. But our respective beliefs were obviously different. I believe that the human soul is eternal and not destroyed by the deterioration of the body. This belief is well supported by the assertion of the Apostle Paul in the Christian scriptures, when he says, " . . . though outwardly we are wasting away, yet inwardly we are being renewed day by day" (II Corinthians 4:16).

I believe that dementia requires a different pastoral care understanding and approach. We have become, even in the spiritual realm, a people who tend to believe only what we can see with our two eyes. Yet on the other hand, God and love are believed in profoundly by millions, yet we can see neither. Though a person's soul experience may not be evident to my observation, is it any less real? If we think so, we as human beings are a very arrogant lot, for the relationship of a person with God is difficult for anyone to determine or define. I have discovered that people with dementia need not change for us; we must change our attitudes toward them so that we can view human life in all its ages and conditions.

As I thought about this clergy person's remark, it became apparent to me that the response is not rare although it is seldom voiced so clearly. Seminary students study abstract ideas about God and are taught how to relate them in abstract ways to cognitively intact persons. This process of conveying the love of God abstractly is irrelevant and unworkable with those who are cognitively impaired.

The end result of my collision with the left-brained value system of religion and spirituality involves questioning how the essences of life and of God may be communicated to those affected by dementia. This leads to the question, "What is dementia?"

WHAT IS DEMENTIA?

Advances in technology and the resultant longer life spans in this century lead to a growing number of people affected by the diseases of aging. According to Alzheimer's Canada, over 300,000 people are affected by Alzheimer's Disease (AD). This number can be multiplied by ten times for the United States. The term dementia is used to describe significant, progressive losses in mental ability, usually but not always in the elderly. Symptoms of dementia include impairment in judgment, thinking, memory and learning as well as possible changes in personality, mood and behavior.

The typical forgetfulness that many of us associate with normal aging is called Benign Sensient Forgetfulness (BS). This forgetfulness is caused by stress, fatigue and an overload of information. Dementia, of which AD constitutes 60-75 percent of the cases, is not a normal part of aging. It is the result of a disease process. At this point in time AD is ultimately terminal. Other types of dementia are largely the result of strokes and more rare neurological diseases.

The time period between onset and total disability from AD ranges from 3 to 20 years. This is part of the reason that a diagnosis brings such dread. With a fairly healthy body, an affected person may live many years while the family copes with erosive changes in personality. There is a pervasive sense of helplessness, and sometimes hopelessness as they watch the progressive demise.

Medical science has not as yet discovered the exact reasons for AD, whether it is due to environmental or genetic factors or a combination of several factors, but one thing is very certain, AD is pervasive in the aging population. With the inclusion of the baby boom generation into the senior category, there will be a tremendous increase in this disruptive societal problem.

NEW UNDERSTANDINGS ABOUT SPIRITUALITY AND AD

One of the exciting discoveries of my studies was creation-centered theology which opened vistas of new understanding of how God and life is experienced. Matthew Fox (1983) is one of the well-known proponents of creation-centered theology, and from his vast writings I have learned that the holy and sacred are experienced and expressed in much broader ways than merely through the cognitive faculty. It is also experienced and expressed through the senses. As the reader becomes familiar with his approach to spirituality, its applicability to ministry with the cognitively impaired becomes apparent.

People do not consist of intellect and memory alone. Thomas Moore (1994) in his book, *The Care of the Soul* was also instrumental in helping me to think differently about the relationship of dementia and spirituality. He courageously looks at reality in a different way. Moore views life from a wellness model rather than the traditional pathological medical model.

Rather than thinking about the person affected by dementia as needing to be "fixed," primarily by drug therapies, the chaplain asks about the yearnings of the soul. For example, a lady in my ministry context was quite aggressive and at times violent, but when music was sung to her, she immediately became calm and even happy. As the patient's past interests, hobbies and other pertinent background become known, the needs of the person can be better fulfilled through natural means, rather than immediate resort to drugs alone. The effects of being in nature is often reported to me by family members as having a calming effect on their loved ones.

My experience with people affected by dementia shows me that what nourishes the mind is not necessarily the same as what nourishes the soul. The cognitively impaired still have emotions, imagination, a will and moral awareness far into the disease process. Feelings retain importance and influence long beyond the time when they can be understood or articulated. These aspects of emotions and imagination are the vital wellsprings from which we experience life's meaning. How can we abandon these people in our ministry of God unless we have a very limited understanding of how God is experienced?

As a chaplain in a Catholic health facility, I have become a strong believer in whole-person care. We are mysteriously interdependent and intertwined beings of physical, mental and spiritual aspects. My ministry is enriched by belief in creation-centered theology and by my conviction that new paradigms of ministry require a major shift in understanding how the brain functions. These were the central thrust of my Master's thesis in Theological Studies at St. Stephen's College. The book version of this thesis is titled *Forget Me Not: The Spiritual Care of People with Alzheimers.*

The article titled "Ministry Without a Future" by Thomas St. James O'Connor (1992) also fuelled my inquiry. The integration of his work with Fox (1983) and Moore (1994) suggests new ways of thinking about persons affected by dementia that are more optimistic than those commonly held in our culture. His optimism is based on a different model of aging than the "over the hill" variety. How could the spiritual needs of those suffering from AD be better addressed if we took a different look?

I believe this research can lead to a higher quality of life for those with dementia as well as for the family members and other caregivers. Although dementia is highly disruptive and currently incurable, it can be approached realistically with hope. This does not in any way deny the loss and grief which lies in the wake of this tragic condition.

A PERSONAL ENCOUNTER OF THE FIRST KIND

I have a multifaceted interest in the area of spiritual care and dementia. My maternal grandmother suffered from progressive dementia for 20 years, commonly referred to in those days as "hardening of the arteries." My questions as a young person were set in the context of confused feelings as I saw my grandmother's ability to communicate change before my eyes. I felt helpless to reach her in the usual verbal manner in the later years and couldn't imagine that there might have been other ways to connect with her. I was puzzled about how her body and soul might be interconnected.

I can not clearly determine how intimately connected my call into ministry was with this experience with dementia, but a linkage certainly exists. I was determined that my ministry would address this concern; my studies helped me create a new model of ministry for helping the cognitively impaired.

How and when do family members and caregivers seek spiritual care? They initially seek information about medical implications, long term care options and practical aspects of dealing with AD. Deeper questions surface after these practical elements have been addressed. Family members are troubled about relationship issues, about whether or not the person they knew and loved is "still in there." If so, what can be done for them? Are there ways to enrich their lives beyond diversionary activities and entertainment? Are there ways to re-establish or maintain connectedness? Has their loved one forgotten any notion of God? Can they still experience God? Chaplains can assist families with these questions, helping them understand how persons experience God beyond the intellect. This is a foundational first step for the chaplain if the spiritual care of people with dementia is to become effective and meaningful.

I believe the cognitively impaired offer unique care and ministry opportunities. Since AD creates an inner wilderness for the affected person, the chaplain must learn to be flexible, creative and concrete. It means that ministers must access both the left and right sides of their brain for ideas and communication pathways. It means accepting and being sensitive to other divergent views, which may include inaccurate memories and feelings of abandonment. It means adapting to unpredictable and unconscious outbursts. Grief and depression are common elements for both the person affected by dementia and their families.

Chaplains, as they come to embrace this area of ministry, can address the often heard statement, "You needn't bother visiting Mary, she won't remember anyway." These poignant words express the feelings of hopelessness and pointlessness that many feel. Chaplains can have a significant input in changing this opinion as they educate caregivers about the meaning of their visits, about the importance of living and valuing each moment of life. By appreciating each moment, we dynamically increase our perception of what is really valuable. A future remembering is not the goal of a visit.

This is an age when busyness is the catch phrase that describes how so many of us see our lives. Much of our society at some level realizes the unhealthiness of this mind set because we sense we are missing an essential reason of living. Strangely enough, it has been in the lives of those affected by dementia that I have learned the lesson of valuing the moment. I have noted how those affected by dementia recognize and appreciate the "little things" of life. One individual with dementia examined with infinite detail the petals of some roses I brought as a central symbol for a hymn sing. I had to question when I had last taken such interest in what God had placed in my life. Had I stopped lately to smell the roses along the way?

DEMENTIA IS A HARSH WINTER

The seasonal changes as we experience them in Canada is a central symbol of life with dementia. I speak of dementia as "a harsh winter." Canadians and many Americans who live in northern climates understand this phrase because there are times in the darkness of winter when we feel the light will never return again. We need hope for the journey as desperately as we need a cure for AD.

Chaplains have a vital role to play in providing hope for families because we have the expertise to address issues of meaning and faith that arise so naturally when the world is turned upside down. One writer (Rosenblatt, 1998) powerfully described his experience with his mother when he says, ". . . in a way, the disease (Alzheimers) demonstrates the essential incomprehensibility of the human mind by reducing it to a puzzle." As family members witness their loved one become a "puzzle," well prepared chaplains can explore with them what this means and how to cope with this reality. They can help families embrace the ever deepening mystery of their loved one, rather than seeking to solve the "puzzle."

But in addition, the image of dementia as the experience of winter symbolically highlights the stripping away of inhibitions experienced by persons with AD. Our inhibitions hide the essence of our real selves. The cognitively intact tend to use masks or inhibitions to prevent society from seeing the real person. The masks are like the summer's growth, obscuring what is inside. Often when someone affected by dementia speaks of how they really feel, we smile with them because the truth of what we feel is so openly expressed. Those affected by dementia help us to discover, to see farther and gain new perspectives about authenticity. Becoming more real would make our lives more healthy.

Those with dementia have taught me how to remove myself from the role of chaplain or minister, to be more myself in pure authenticity. They are not impressed with my degrees or my ordination. This understanding became very evident also to the well-known theologian Henri Nouwen, author of many books on spirituality. He left a highly prestigious university position and entered the life of L'Arche, a community of the mentally challenged founded by Jean Vanier.

Nouwen's book (1989), *In the Name of Jesus: Reflections of Christian Leadership,* describes the human being who is really lovable as very basic and real. My ministry with AD has taught me that God is best communicated through the real me. In this light, those affected by dementia have revealed for me the paradoxical nature of ministry for God. They have highlighted in a way like no book could, that the hiddenness of God is largely my own making. They have highlighted in the deepest manner that God is found in the weak and the often perceived unacceptable amongst us. This realization is extremely humbling and life transforming. In actuality, those affected by dementia are our greatest teachers.

In this winter image of dementia, where we look most of all for the familiar and warm face, I have discovered that ministry is only as good as the minister who values presence as the core element of love and care. Christian theology is built on the concept of the incarnation, God-with-us. When the chaplain values the importance of his/her presence and is not concerned about accomplishing something, the meaningfulness of ministry increases dramatically.

THE MYRIAD OF COMMUNICATION PATHWAYS

So, how do we convey the love of God and others? When we research the ways in which we communicate, it is startling to realize that 80-90 percent of our communication is nonverbal. I believe the core reason our society has struggled to value the lives of those suffering from dementia is largely due to our overemphasis on the verbal and cognitive. We have become "the information age" and knowledge is prized above everything else.

If a deeper and wider experience of the world can be realized through a greater awareness and appreciation of touch, music, presence, love, smell, color, play, pets, humor and nature, what could this mean in the lives of those affected by dementia? Spirituality must be understood in a wider context then the intellect, in the realm of our bodies and emotions. What would this broader understanding of spirituality mean? It would mean that we might re-vision and balance ministry concerns to care for those with dementia with the same energy and enthusiasm as the general population. It could conceivably revitalize the respect of faith communities that primarily reach the young, cognitively intact and upwardly mobile.

Music is a central means of communication with those affected by dementia. It is rhythm and rhythm is the most primal connection to existence. Rhythm was the first sound we all heard when we were conceived in our mother's womb; her heartbeat. Because long term memories are the last to leave in the process of dementia, music is also one of the last communication pathways that reach the soul.

Music, so powerfully affecting our emotions and our memories, is also a central means of experiencing and expressing the sacred. This does not mean that chaplains have to play an instrument or be great singers; they can use taped music and organize volunteers to provide this ministry. Research (Bailey, 1993) has demonstrated, however, that live music has a more immediate effect than that which is taped.

ETHICAL CONCERNS AND DEMENTIA

Another of the important ways that a chaplain offers ministry with those affected by dementia and their families is in the area of ethics. The chaplain has much to offer in addressing the social justice issues of the elderly. The elderly and especially those affected by dementia have been ostracized in our society and sidelined by their age and abilities. We are not comfortable in our "doing" society with those who are simply " being." The dilemma of valuing the aged is with us.

Chaplains have the unique opportunity to be a bridge between the health care system and the community. They can address the public by asking why health care dollars are predominately directed towards acute systems. Only the leftovers of our budgets are given to chronic care facilities. Chaplains can speak to the public about the unethical ways we donate money for the "glamour" diseases which affect few people and those in the "prime" of life, while research and treatment efforts in dementia are simply maintained with the least possible expenditure in time, money and expertise.

Chaplains can address how society has changed in the past decades as regards attitudes toward caregiving. We have become an individualistic society due to mobility and the entry of women into the work force. Yet, women are still the major AD caregivers. We need to address how the allocation of caregiving dollars must become wider to include community involvement, as well as respite and daycare opportunities. The chaplain has opportunity to address all of these ethical concerns.

GRIEF AND DEMENTIA:
THE MEANING MAKING PROCESS

Chaplains can also address the questions concerning "meaning" which are part of the grief process. With AD individuals, chaplains can assist the grief concerning their many losses by validating their feelings over and over again. This, again, is the valuable ministry of the moment.

Families often raise questions as to why this is happening. Sometimes they ask, "How can a loving God permit this to happen?" This does not imply that chaplains give easy answers, but rather that they assist people to image God as companion, a supportive and understanding friend in the midst of senselessness.

This ministry interjects the faithfulness of God into the experience of unpredictably and frightening months and years of degenerative disease. In the midst of forgetfulness and the loss of control, the chaplain represents a God who never forgets us (cf. Isaiah 49:15).

I conduct at the request of the Edmonton Alzheimer Society an annual Alzheimer Awareness Candlelight Service at the Edmonton General Hospital. This is a wonderful opportunity to regularly remind caregivers and families that in the midst of difficulties and grief, God is the Constant One who can be relied upon. One of the features of this service has been the playing of Pachebel's Canon while Psalm 136 is read, a psalm which repeatedly states that God's steadfast love is present in all the eventualities of life. In the service, we light seven candles. These seven represent those who have died of AD, those who live with it, their families, caregivers, those who do research, volunteers and the public. The verbal response recited at the lighting of each candle is, "Come, let us walk in the light of peace, hope, love, trust, faith, belief and truth."

Hope in the face of dementia means taking the Christian scripture of Philippians 4:8 more seriously. "Finally . . . whatever things are true, whatever is right, whatever is pure think about such things." The writer speaks of thinking not on the negative, but on what is positive. With dementia we tend to look exclusively on what is lost. What is lost needs to be recognized and grieved, but a more balanced perspective is needed. A balanced perspective leads to a hope based on the ongoing possibilities for better care that lies with what is left. A more positive outlook will lead to greater enthusiasm to support the people affected, to support of the families, for educating the public, lobbying governments and encouraging research. Thinking on these things will bring light into our darkness.

This style of ministry fits into the more recent grief research. This research moves away from the stages-of-grief model to one of meaning-making and understanding the choices and options available to those who are involved in long-term grieving for family members with AD. These family members do pass through prescribed stages of grief when they are dealing with a disease process that can last two decades.

The AD experience teaches that life is not neatly experienced in a linear manner. No, life is lived more in a spiral or labyrinth modality. It is living through, embracing and expressing all the feelings we have, finding meaning and hope in the journey through grief. This is the ministry of chaplains.

The research project of Pratt, Schmall, Wright and Cleland entitled, "Burden and Coping Strategies of Caregivers of Alzheimer's Patients" which investigated the situations of 240 subjects, discovered that the two most important external coping mechanisms were spiritual support and an extended family. Spiritual support was described as finding the meaning of the situation and in clarifying expectations. The chaplain can play an important role here in reframing expectations, and neutralizing potential stressors by seeking positive attributes.

The chaplain can help the family and other care givers by modelling and educating them in a healthy spirituality that accepts limitations, hope in the face of suffering, unconditional love for its own sake, and dispelling any punitive images of God.

In conclusion, ministry with those who are cognitively impaired presents us with a surprising paradox. As we open ourselves to embracing them as wholly worthwhile and valuable persons that need motivated and loving care, they expel us from our intellectual theological boxes. In the process, they introduce us to a God who is also dancing and laughing in the bizarre places where chaos reigns.

Certainly, "they are the forgotten ones who can teach us the numinous quality of all of creation which we forget is there. They are the symbol of the 'holy' otherness, a revelation of the hidden face of God" (Pratt 1985).

REFERENCES

Doka, K., Davidson, J. (Eds). 1997. *Living with grief when illness is prolonged.* Taylor and Francis Publishing, Hospice Foundation of America.

Everett, Debbie. 1996. *Forget me not: The spiritual care of people with Alzheimers.* Edmonton, Alberta, Canada: Inkwell Press.

Fox, Matthew. 1983. *Original blessing.* Santa Fe, New Mexico: Bear and Co.

Lucanne Magill Bailey. 1993. "The effects of live music versus tape recorded music on hospitalized cancer patients." *The Journal of Music Therapy,* 3(1),17-28.

Moore, Thomas. 1994. *Care of the soul.* New York: Harper Perennial.

Nouwen, Henri. 1989. *In the name of Jesus: Reflections of Christian leadership.* New York, Crossroads.

O'Connor, Thomas St. James. 1992. Ministry without a future. *The Journal of Pastoral Care,* 46(1), Spring.

Pratt, C.C. et al. 1985. Burden and coping strategies of caregiving of Alzheimer's patients and family relations. *Family Relations,* 34, 27-33.

Rosenblatt, Roger. January 12, 1998. The Long Disease. *Time Magazine.*

All Biblical quotations are from the New International Version (1973). International Bible Society, Zondervan Corporation, Grand Rapids, Michigan.

Assuring Professional Pastoral Care for Every Nursing Home Resident

Bethany Knight, MA

SUMMARY. Ministry to persons in nursing homes is built on two mandates: ". . . He has sent me to bring good news to the oppressed, to bind up the brokenhearted, to proclaim liberty to the captives, and release to the prisoners; . . . to comfort all who mourn . . ." (Isaiah 61:1-3). The federal government provides the second: "Quality of Life. A facility must care for its residents in a manner and in an environment that promotes maintenance or enhancement of each resident's quality of life" (OBRA '87, Guidance to Surveyors in Long Term Care Facilities, Code of Federal Regulations, Health Care Financing Administration, 1995, section 483.15, F240). This article discusses both the religious and the U.S. political history of caring for the old and frail. It concludes by describing political efforts in one state to increase the quality of that care and pastoral efforts to support the nursing assistants in long-term care facilities. *[Article copies available for a fee from The Haworth Document Delivery Service: 1-800-342-9678. E-mail address: getinfo@haworthpressinc.com]*

Wrestling with end of life concerns is the central spiritual issue facing residents and staff of long term care facilities. What can chaplains do to focus resources and time on this great ache, thus fulfilling the charges of both Isaiah and the federal government? One can argue that Church and State agree on the need for attention to end of life issues. The language of Congress's Omnibus Reconciliation Act of 1987, OBRA '87 quoted above is simply a secular restatement of Isaiah.

Bethany Knight is CNA President, Northern Knights, Glover, VT.

[Haworth co-indexing entry note]: "Assuring Professional Pastoral Care for Every Nursing Home Resident." Knight, Bethany. Co-published simultaneously in *Journal of Health Care Chaplaincy* (The Haworth Pastoral Press, an imprint of The Haworth Press, Inc.) Vol. 8, No. 1/2, 1999, pp. 89-107; and: *Spiritual Care for Persons with Dementia: Fundamentals for Pastoral Practice* (ed: Larry VandeCreek) The Haworth Pastoral Press, an imprint of The Haworth Press, Inc., 1999, pp. 89-107. Single or multiple copies of this article are available for a fee from The Haworth Document Delivery Service [1-800-342-9678, 9:00 a.m. - 5:00 p.m. (EST). E-mail address: getinfo@haworthpressinc.com].

Even in our death denying and defying culture, once one crosses the nursing home threshold it is hard to run or hide from mortality. According to the American Health Care Association (1998), the nation's trade organization for nursing homes, the typical nursing home patient is a widow in her late eighties with multiple medical problems, surrounded by strangers and living in an unfamiliar setting.

"Am I going to die? Is there a heaven or hell?" she worries, turning to the woman at her bedside for answers. That woman, a certified nursing assistant with, at most, a high school education, is staring down questions of her own, "What should I say? How come every one I touch dies? How much longer can I work here, with all this death?"

In the introduction to their epoch work, *The Nursing Home in American Society* (1985), Colleen Johnson and Leslie Grant write that nursing homes have been commonly referred to as "houses of death" and "warehouses for the dying."

So profound is this confrontation with the finite nature of life, it has now been identified as the number one reason nursing assistants quit their jobs. For her master's thesis as a graduate student at Appalachian State University, in 1991, V. Beverly Nickles studied why nurses' aides in a three-state region quit their jobs. The overwhelming reason stated by aides at exit interviews: death.

More recently, Richard Hoffman (1997), writing in *Nursing Assistant Monthly,* stated that one of the major problems driving nursing assistant turnovers is that they "are put into relationships with residents who die and there is seldom any acknowledgment of the grief they feel." Nationally, that turnover is 101 percent.

Both of these studies echo what aides know and what they will tell you if asked. At the beginning of this decade, I created and conducted 50 workshops across Vermont, exclusively for nurses' aides, entitled *Recharge Your Batteries.* A section of the workshop, designed to bring the group together, required participants to list, individually, the 10 best parts of the job and the 10 worst. These lists were then read aloud and compared. Having worked as a long term care ombudsman for two years, I expected to hear the worst part of the job would be working short staffed, the heavy lifting, the pay. But hundreds of nurses' aides set me straight, answering simply, "death."

All societies and cultures have dealt with illness and death, some better than others. Our European ancestors were well aware of the spiritual needs of the sick and dying. Indeed, the first hospitals, infirmaries and hospices were built by the Church, with the alter the central feature, much like the prominence of today's nurses' stations.

In Roman times, people always took care of their own kin at home when they were sick. The three exceptions the community was willing to care for were soldiers, gladiators and slaves, because they were valuable assets to the economy. Paupers died.

GREATER THE VICTIM'S MISERY, THE GREATER ATTENDANT'S VALUE AND MERIT

In their comprehensive 1975 work, *The Hospital: A Social and Architectural History,* John Thompson and Grace Goldin outlined the history of caregiving in the Western world. The first Christians sought to perform "care work," and based it on carrying out Matthew 25:35-36, the six acts of mercy mentioned there: "For I was hungry, and you gave me food, I was thirsty and you gave me something to drink, I was a stranger and you welcomed me, I was naked and you gave me clothing, I was sick and you took care of me, I was in prison and you visited me."

Later, Christians added a seventh act of mercy, burying the dead, referencing the Book of Tobit 1:16-17: "In the time of Shalmaneser, I did many acts of charity for my fellow countrymen: I shared my food with the hungry and provided clothes for the naked. If I saw the dead body of any man of my race lying outside the wall of Ninevah, I buried it."

For 1000 years, the motivation of Christian charitable institutions was shaped by the seven mercies. St. Chrysostom said, "If there were no poor, the greater part of your sins would not be removed; they are the healers of your wounds." In fact, the victim's degree of misery enhanced his value and merit to the attendant.

Pilgrims became the first sick individuals to require care outside the private home, because they were not near their families, to whom normally this duty would fall. Undertaking a long journey, always a form of penance, pilgrims were probably in a weakened or ill condition to begin with. Travel was tough, food strange and/or insufficient. Ancient documents indicate that, as early as the 5th century, if one wanted a private room, he or she had to pay extra.

The matron Fabiola, in fourth century Rome, turned her home into a refuge for the sick, and helped build a hospice in Rome for pilgrims from Africa. And 800 years later, St. Elizabeth of Hungary, took the afflicted into her own castle, and said, "How well it is for us that thus we bathe and cover our Lord!"

In Syria in AD 370, St. Basil opened his hospital and leprosarium. One hundred years later, the Hospice of Turmanin was built in Syria, on the main road between Antioch and Qalat-simon. An inn for pilgrims, it was intentionally shaped like the cross Jesus was crucified upon, with four wings. The campus included a church, an administrative building and a convent or inn for dispensing hospitality to pilgrims.

At the monastery of St. Gall in Switzerland, a major care center opened in 817 was staffed by 110 monks and even had a bloodletting house.

Guiding these homes of Christian charity was the Rule of St. Benedict, "Before all things and above all things care must be taken of the sick, so that they may be served in very deed as Christ himself; for he said, 'I was sick and ye visited me.' Let there be assigned a special attendant who is God fearing, diligent and careful."

The Religious of Cluny, France, two centuries later in 1000 AD, built monasteries with infirmaries. The arrangement was an open ward with a central chapel and alter, so the sick could see the daily Mass and most importantly, the host lifted during the service. This cross design also aided in ventilation and supervision.

The Hospital of Santa Maria Nuova served the poor of Florence, Italy in the 15th and 16th centuries, with two cross-designed wards, one for men and one for women.

At the Hospital de Santa Cruz at Toledo, Spain, a splinter from the real cross was purportedly built into the building. The hospital was built on a regal scale, for "people for whom one could expect no returns, people who today's society regards as a burden. . . . The incurably sick had the love of the people and the royal favor, for heaven was open to them. So, the hospital becomes a Golgotha, and the sick become the precious possession of the community" (p. 34).

By the 1700s, modesty and morality began to drive the need for privacy within the institution, and away from huge wards.

The Reformation had a powerful impact on the existing models of care. A new hospital arose, and the Crown and not the Church, was the sponsor. The Bourgeoisie, not the Church, paid the bills. The goal was to make cities a healthier place to live, creating a system of social aid.

The order was issued in London in 1569 that the aged, sick, lame and blind should be sent to St. Bart's or St. Thomas's hospitals. Gone was the assumption that any 'poor object' might be the Lord Jesus Christ in disguise.

What had once been paid for through charitable offerings was now compulsory. All citizens were responsible for paying a tax to cover the expenses of caring for the poor of their parish, including the costs of bringing them back to the parish from points afar. If the tax was unpaid, the scofflaw was imprisoned.

Around 1755, Europe marked the end of the era of the palatial hospital, with the public sentiment being the poor should be kept in poor circumstances. It soon became too complicated to return indigent poor to their home parish, and the hospitals' admission policy was simply, "whatever corner of the world they come from, they come without restriction." This no-discrimination policy became the founding central policy of the American hospital movement, when this nation's first hospitals opened their doors in Philadelphia, Boston and New York City. People of means were still cared for at home, and, as in the old country, hospitals were still basically for visitors, paupers and the insane.

THE NURSING HOME:
FASHIONED FROM THE HOSPITAL'S RIB

In this fledgling country, local governments took responsibility for the poor, mentally ill, blind and sick, not only through taxes but also through a variety of self-supporting institutional programs such as almshouses, orphanages and poor farms. It seems America's solution to poverty and other social problems has been institutionalization. And whenever possible, government has tried to make these institutions self-supporting, hence the establishment of the poor farm.

Colleen Johnson and Leslie Grant (1985) traced the origins of nursing homes in the United States, in *The Nursing Home in American Society*. Between 1910 and 1970, the proportion of the elderly residing in institutions increased 267 percent! In 1910, only 80,000 older Americans lived in mental institutions or almshouses. By 1970, with almshouses all closed, 1.1 million older Americans lived in institutions, close to 73 percent in nursing homes and 10 percent in mental institutions.

By some estimates, the number of nursing home beds doubled between 1963 and 1973. In 1985, there are two to three times more nursing homes than general hospitals and consequently more patient beds and days in nursing homes than hospitals. What happened in the United States during these 60 years to push so many elders in institutions?

In the early 1920s, less than 0.6 percent of those over 65 lived in what were called "charitable private homes for the aged," operated by immigrant self help groups and various religious groups. By 1930, more people of this age group lived in mental hospitals than in the poor houses and homes for the aged, combined.

What changed was the introduction of the Social Security Act in 1935, providing retirees with money to use for their care. This Act also made grants to the states, and thus made the state responsible for care of the helpless. Interestingly enough, this money could not be used in institutional settings, per the Act. This policy was designed to keep institutions from growing. However, it was eventually altered, and money could be used to pay for care delivered in private, but not public, institutions. After World War II, public poorhouses evolved into nursing homes, as they were primarily full of old people. By the 1960s, what we now know as the long term care institution was born, with the creation of Medicaid.

Two other government acts propelled the rapid growth of the nation's nursing homes into mini-sub acute care hospitals; the Hill-Burton Act, which provided federal dollars to nursing homes if they met certain medical acute care requirements, and the deinstitutionalization of mental hospitals. In the majority of cases, the elderly ex-mental patients eventually ended up living in nursing homes, unable to function or find support outside the institutional environment.

Nursing homes became a facility, not much like home.

WHAT DO RESIDENTS WANT?

From a resident's standpoint, when asked what is the most important factor when living in a nursing home, the answer is uniform: "good staff." The Nursing Home Community Coalition and the Coalition of Institutionalized Aged and Disabled of NYC have conducted focus groups of nursing home residents. They have characterized a good relationship between residents and staff as requiring staff who show compassion and kindness, treat you like a human being, work together with you when providing care, are well trained, meet your individual needs, with a good disposition, talk to you in a pleasant and respectful manner and can develop a trusting relationship where humor can take place.

If the key to a successful nursing home stay is staff, but staffs leave in record numbers each year because they can't deal with death, why aren't facilities helping staff deal with death? In other words, why isn't there a full time chaplain in all 12,000 nursing homes in this country?

To answer this question, we need to remember the origins of the nursing home industry, its genesis.

THE MEDICAID PROGRAM: AMERICA'S DEFAULT LONG TERM CARE INSURANCE

In the late 1960s, through a marriage of state and federal governments, and with the blessing of President Lyndon Johnson and his Great Society, Medicaid was born. This state-federal program was designed to pay for the medical care of the indigent. Now, 30 plus years later, it is the primary insurance for long term care in the United States. Medicaid pays 68 percent of the nation's nursing home bills, close to $31 billion annually (American Health Care Association, 1998). And remember, this is a bill government never anticipated.

According to Bruce Vladeck (1981), who wrote *Unloving Care,* and later went on to become the head of the Health Care Financing Administration, "The history of public policy toward nursing homes is largely a by-product of broader social welfare legislation, but in a tangential fashion. The history is like describing the opening of the American West from the perspective of mules; they were certainly there, and the epochal events were certainly critical to mules, but hardly anyone was paying very much attention to them at the time."

From this quite-by-accident beginning, nursing homes and long-term care Medicaid have evolved into one of the most complex, paper heavy programs in human history. Providers of care maintain they are the country's most heavily regulated industry, even more so than nuclear power. Virtually nothing happens in a nursing home that doesn't appear in a state or federal regulation. The number of hours between snacks and meals served, the number of feet between beds, the water temperature for washing laundry, dishes and people are all set by regulation.

Working in this kind of proscribed environment, natural human instincts and behaviors change. Creativity is not sought or rewarded. Consequently, the individual with insight or vision isn't typically sought, hired or valued. What nursing homes tend to attract are managers who like routine and predictability. Administrators who make a career in the nursing home are often creatures of habit, repeating the Monday routine the other five days of the week. If Medicaid pays most of the bills (in Vermont, almost 70 percent of the patients are Medicaid), the thinking goes, why do anything for patients that Medicaid doesn't reimburse?

For more than 10 years, I directed the Vermont Health Care Association, the state's trade organization for nursing and residential care facilities, affiliated with the American Health Care Association. It provides continuing education for the staff of member facilities. Trade association executives know the trick in sponsoring and successful seminars or workshops is appealing to the right motivator of member behavior. Even Pavlov's dog knew that there has to be a reason to do anything! I still recall the poorly attended workshops we offered on massage, the value of the human touch, body mechanics and how to avoid injury on the job. Because Medicaid hadn't mentioned these subjects, it was as if they didn't exist.

I found that to get an educational program on the nursing home administrator's radar screen, one needed to relate it to a new law or regulation, federal or state, and use that ace motivator, Fear. Any program that played to an administrator's fear of receiving a deficiency on an inspection survey sold out. Like the rest of the species, long-term care management is concerned with safety and security. Nobody wants trouble.

So what has Medicaid or any branch of the federal government said about death in nursing homes? Unfortunately, nothing. And herein lies the answer to why chaplains are not employed by every nursing home, why spirituality and death are overlooked.

Curiously, the Medicare program does address religious needs of patients, when it mandates that spiritual care be part of the interdisciplinary hospice team. Hospice programs without provision for spiritual care are not certified, i.e., receive no Medicare reimbursement. With this strong, fear motivator, all of this country's certified Medicare hospices have spiritual care available for patients who die at home.

VERMONT'S EXPERIENCE

Given that as many people die in a nursing home as home, it seems incredible that the law and its rules are silent on helping residents and staff of long term care facilities deal with death. In Vermont, we began introducing the hospice concept into nursing homes at the opening of this decade. The hospice community did not initially embrace nursing facilities, stating that this unique approach to death could not be offered in a nursing home. Gradually, relationships were built between hospice providers–the home health agencies–and nursing homes.

The attitudes and needs expressed by nurses' aides at my workshops in the early 1990s caused me to pursue the creation of death education for staff.

Many nursing home administrators told me directly they did not want to talk about death, that it was too depressing, and if I wanted to offer useful educational programs, I should focus on recruiting and retaining staff. I shared my data about the direct linkage between death and aides quitting work, but no one wanted to hear it. The chair of the Association's education committee actually forbid any workshops on death at our annual convention, stating, "We want to get together to have a good time." In spite of this denial, a workshop was offered on death, called Celebration of Life. It received the most powerful evaluations from participants our Association had ever recorded. Direct care staff were starved for knowledge and permission to be sad. No one had told them it was appropriate and natural to cry when they had to say good bye. Instead, they had been told, "Don't get too close to a patient, use no terms of endearment, please."

INTRODUCING MEMORIAL SERVICES
INTO NURSING HOMES

Buoyed by my own primary research on the subject, I was further inspired to help create a program to minister to the spiritual needs of staff and residents of nursing facilities by an article written by Lea

Pardue (1991). This included my writing a book of daily devotions for nurses' aides, pursued and received credentialing as a licensed local pastor within the United Methodist Church, and licensure as a nurses' aide.

Pardue reported on a study conducted under the auspices of the Gerontological Society of America's Student Fellowship Program in Applied Gerontology. Semi-structured interviews were conducted with resident council members from three nursing homes in northern North Carolina. While the essence of the study was that residents and clergy do not perceive the spiritual needs of residents similarly, I was struck by another finding. "Residents felt that they needed regular involvement with others sharing similar religious beliefs both in worship services and in individual witnessing" (p. 13).

Pardue's evidence that group religious experiences in nursing homes are important to residents led me to pilot a memorial service at Berlin Health Rehabilitation Services, Berlin, VT. With the BHRC's activities director, a service was designed to carefully and respectfully broach the subject of death.

Spending time with nurses' aides, I had learned that most facilities followed a similar protocol when death came visiting:

- doors to other residents' rooms were closed, with and without explanation;
- the body was covered and moved into a storage area, designed for other purposes, often a supply closet or the boiler room;
- facilities generally waited until darkness to have the body taken from the building, using a rear door;
- residents and other staff learned of the death as they learned most news of facility life–by chance and through casual conversation.

After conducting a few memorial services at BHRS, I saw the tremendous value of such a ritual for not only all staff, but for the other residents. Mildred, a frail former school teacher bent nearly double by osteoporosis, looked up at me one afternoon from her wheelchair following our service. "Will you talk about me when my time comes?"

"Yes," I promised. "I have so much to say!"

"Good," she said, and wheeled away.

I believe a great fear associated with dying in a nursing home is the worry that no one will notice. Aides report that after a death occurred and the body is moved, able residents routinely pass by the room and peek in, to confirm the loss and the truth.

Why not put a rose on the bed? Or a sash on the door, connoting a great soul has passed? Like Tobit, we should not pass a body without properly tending to it. To create rituals and protocols to honestly and gently inform staff and other residents someone has died is most assuredly an act of mercy.

At about this time, Rev. Regis Cummings, a visiting chaplain at BHRS and a deacon at St. Augustine's church in Montpelier, Vermont, was named by Vermont Governor Howard Dean to the Board of Examiners for Nursing Home Administrators, the state licensing board. Selected to be the public representative on the Board, Rev. Cummings was sent to several national conferences on the Omnibus Reconciliation Act of 1987, the most sweeping federal reform of the nursing home industry. This major piece of legislation, which mandated such basics as completion of a minimum of 75 hours of nurses' aide training before new aides can touch a patient, also addressed issues influencing the quality of life and care in nursing homes. Upon returning from one such conference, Rev. Cummings contacted me.

"I've been visiting nursing homes for more than 15 years as a Catholic chaplain," he told me, "there is such a need for ministering to the spirit, among residents and staff. I go to these workshops on quality of life, which we know means ministry to the spirit. Yet, no one seems to know how to speak about it, let alone deliver it." From our own vantage points, Rev. Cummings and I came together and decided to define and improve quality of life in nursing homes.

Working with a dedicated group of extraordinarily talented volunteers, we established the Foundation for Compassionate Care (FCC), a not-for-profit corporation which considers ways of strengthening nursing homes, especially staff and residents' morale in matters broadly pertaining to spirituality.

The FCC developed a series of focused seminars, entitled "Rediscovering, Exploring and Awakening the Spiritual Dimension of Quality Care in Nursing Homes." Our Foundation's team includes (in addition to Rev. Cummings and myself) a registered nurse who works in a home for the aged and is the co-founder of a cancer support group and spiritual journey group; a theologian in ancient civilizations and religions, who is also an educator and author; an administrator and author who is also an elementary school principal; and a lawyer who is also a teacher and chaplain in crisis intervention and advocacy.

Our workshop series is six hours long, held in shorter segments over different days, at the convenience of the facility. It is designed for all disciplines within the nursing home, as well as volunteers and community members. Following completion of the six hour series, two follow up sessions of three hours each are offered, focusing on implementing specific concepts at the facility, including developing support groups, creating rituals for dealing with death and other losses and recognizing the patient's religious traditions, their significance and meaning.

Beyond offering resources to nursing homes, the Foundation strongly urges the establishment of in-house part-time chaplaincy or a spiritual support position, to assist staff and residents in spiritual matters, and assure the ongoing use of knowledge gained during the workshops.

One important distinction the FCC makes in all its work is to delineate the difference between religion and spirituality: religion is but one form of spirituality, and often co-exists in the same person, with other forms of spirituality.

"The importance and legitimacy of the dimension of human spirituality, as a quality of life issue, is now widely recognized in government, business and law. Especially in an environment such as that of nursing homes, to which residents entrust numerous aspects of their personal lives, it would seem vital to recognize the function of spirituality, in one form or another. While nursing homes are never the primary providers or opportunities for spirituality, neither should nursing homes fail to be sensitive and supportive in this area," said Rev. Cummings, when petitioning Vermont's nursing home inspectors to consider matters spiritual when surveying facilities. In particular, on behalf of the FCC, Rev. Cummings suggested the state require facilities to have death and bereavement policies, and mandate some mention of "spirituality awareness" be provided to nurses' aides in their training.

To date, these suggestions have not been adopted, but the Foundation continues to persevere. A handful of facilities have participated in workshops, though most claim they cannot afford to pay for such education. While a minimal fee is charged, it seems because the club of government does not hang over head, facilities do not appear motivated to seize this profound opportunity. Those that have hosted the FCC series find that staff members are extremely satisfied with the workshops. As one administrator stated, "This is a worthwhile program of 'opening a door' to the spiritual dimensions, with a renewed awareness of the spiritual needs of the patients, caregivers and families."

OMNIBUS RECONCILIATION ACT OF 1987 (OBRA '87): A SPIRITUAL ALLY?

Once OBRA became law, the federal government (Health Care Financing Administration, 1995) wrote the Code of Federal Regulations (CFR) to implement the law. In each state, the Code's chief messengers and enforcers are state nurse inspectors with whom the federal government contracts to survey nursing facilities on an annual, unannounced basis. Within the CFR is a Quality of Life section. The main tag number (the language which a surveyor will cite when finding the facility not in compliance with code) is F240:

> Quality of Life: A facility must care for its residents in a manner and in an environment that promotes maintenance or enhancement of each resident's quality of life.

Other related tags are:

> F241: Dignity: The facility must promote care for residents in a manner and in an environment that maintains or enhances each resident's dignity and respect in full recognition of his or her individuality.

> F242: Self determination and participation: The resident has the right to:

> > 1–choose activities, schedules, and health care consistent with his or her interests, assessments, and plans of care;
> > 2–interact with members of the community both inside and outside the facility; and
> > 3–make choices about aspects of his or her life in the facility that are significant to the resident.

F245: Participation in other activities: A resident has a right to participate in social, religious and community activities that do not interfere with the rights of other residents in the facility.

F246: Accommodation of needs: A resident has a right to reside and receive services in the facility with reasonable accommodations of individual needs and preferences, except when the health or safety of the individual or other residents would be endangered.

A savvy chaplain will ask the nursing facility administrator for the latest state survey report, and check to see if any of these tag numbers are cited. If so, the facility has been put on notice that resident quality of life needs are not being adequately met. This survey deficiency can become the foot in the door for the interested chaplain, that is, an entry point into discussions with the home's management about meeting the spiritual needs of residents.

In the decade since OBRA's controversial implementation, many significant improvements have occurred in the nation's nursing homes, from the viewpoint of residents, regulators, providers and taxpayers alike (The Commonwealth Fund, 1996). Since the institution of OBRA '87 nationally:

- There has been nearly a 50 percent reduction in the use of restraints, freeing 250,000 elderly patients each year.
- There has been a significant increase in the involvement of families and residents in care plan meetings and decisions.
- Psychotropic drug use has dropped by as much as a third.
- Behavior management programs for wandering, aggression, or resisting care have increased by 27 percent.
- The use of toileting programs for incontinence has doubled.
- The use of hearing aids has increased by 30 percent.

Proudly, Vermont (Vermont Agency of Human Services, 1998) boasts the lowest use of physical restraints in the nation, with just 2.84 of our nursing home patients tied up. Twenty of the state's 46 nursing homes use no restraints. One must quickly add that much remains to be done, with regard to reducing the use of chemical restraints, i.e., behavior altering medications.

"Based on my observations and conversations, I would say OBRA has yet to shine within the domain referred to as 'quality of life,'" said DAD Commissioner David Yacovone, a former nursing home administrator (Personal interview 1998). "Defining quality is not a simple task, but that doesn't mean regulators and providers shouldn't strive to do so. Does the greater use of hearing aides improve quality of life? Yes, I think so. But so does a developed hospice program, with attention paid to spiritual needs. The community at large, and particularly the nation's churches, could provide a great service by asking those who live and work in these facilities 'what spiritual needs can we help with?' I understand that it is still fairly common for nursing home patients to die alone, because staff cannot make the time to sit with them."

TWO STUDIES OF DEATH IN VERMONT

Two studies of how Vermonters regard death affirms Commissioner Yacovone's sense that Vermont, and quite certainly, the rest of the nation's nursing homes, has yet to satisfactorily deal with the OBRA mandate called Quality of Life.

Between January and June of 1996, my son Elliot Kaiman and I launched a data collection project with nursing homes, separate and apart from my work with VHCA. Twelve homes volunteered to participate.

Our project was to look at the factors surrounding patient deaths in nursing homes: including average length of stay, age at death and unusual circumstances at time of death. Given that we are amateurs, our research was not scientific. However, the results are still thought provoking, and, more than anything, question provoking. (Thanks to the volunteer efforts of Coleen Condon of Burlington, VT, who compiled our data.)

We surveyed a total of 884 beds. Of the homes reporting, 66 percent of the patients who died were females. About 48 percent of all those who died received hospice-type care. We defined hospice as palliative care, keeping a patient pain free with no extraordinary treatment or left alone. Other results included the average age at death (males = 75.3; females = 88) and the average length of stay (680 days or 1.86 years). About 9 percent of those who died had a significant experience immediately prior to death, including a visit from a son or daughter, an anniversary or birthday. This figure could be much higher because it is highly dependent on the staffs' power of observation.

It was unexpected that almost half of the deaths that occurred in the facilities were classified by staff as hospice-type care. Just five years earlier, the word death and hospice were never uttered in such settings. Of course, the participating facilities were volunteers; they represented less than one third of the state's nursing homes. One must presume that these facilities were collectively more comfortable with the subject of death.

Again, the savvy chaplain can find another place to insert his or her presence in the life of the facility, by talking with the director of nursing about the facility's provision of hospice-type care. This model of care for the dying very much encourages spiritual services, and hence, the involvement of the chaplain.

In 1997, to learn how Vermonters were thinking about the care of the dying, the Vermont Ethics Network, with major support from the Project on Death in America, undertook a series of community forums, entitled Journey's End, in which groups of Vermonters were asked to reflect on their own experiences with such care.

According to the Vermont Department of Health, about 45 percent of Vermonters die in hospital, 24 percent at home and 23 percent in nursing homes.

"Surprisingly, the nursing home as a site for dying was not often mentioned, though about as many Vermonters die there as die at home. The quality of dying in nursing homes was as variable as in hospitals; it could be remembered by survivors with gratitude or with regret. We heard the nursing described as a 'lifeboat,' engendering caring links between strangers. 'Staff was caring, informative, supportive in every way–physical, emotional and spiritual . . . '

And we heard of other nursing homes as 'crowded, lots of confused patients, little privacy,' or of dying patients swept up in inappropriate routines such as mandated 'socialization' in the day rooms. 'Mother was in a four-bed room, the others were moaning and kept wanting to talk to me. I couldn't spend that time quietly with my mother.' "

One of the Vermont Ethics Network (1997) report recommendations calls for "development of hospice-style care in hospitals, nursing homes and congregate residential settings." The report also noted, "spiritual needs are common to all human encounters with serious illness, but become especially prominent as death approaches. Most participants were keenly aware of this."

NATIONAL ASSOCIATION
OF GERIATRIC NURSING ASSISTANTS FOUNDED

As is often the case during times of major social change, many divergent interest groups seem to see the same needs and voice the same concerns at the same time, and cause, in effect, a creative relay. In 1995, two former nurses' aides turned long term care executives founded the National Association of Geriatric Nursing Assistants (NAGNA) in Joplin, Missouri. After more than 6 years as a nurses' aide, Lori Porter had pursued the necessary education and became a nursing home administrator. Lisa Cantrell, also a nurses' aide, had pursued nursing degrees and became a director of nursing in a nursing facility.

With this professional background, these two pioneering women started NAGNA, founded on the guiding principle that not only are nurses' aides the backbone of the nursing home industry, they are its heart and soul as well. Today, more than 12,500 aides are NAGNA members, participating in workshops on professionalism, conquering job stress and burnout, self motivation, turnover reduction and building a winning team.

Ministering to the precious nurses' aide, NAGNA's statement of standards (1996) includes these words all members take to heart:

I am part of a noble profession, rendering a valuable humanitarian service to others who are dependent on me for their personal care. I am a responsible dependable caregiver, and I render my help and assistance to those in my charge as through their lives depended on it, because they do. My standard is The Golden Rule. I render care as I would have it given to me if I were in their place. I am rightfully proud of the work I do because it is a special service and I am a special person. I will seek to use all available resources to increase my knowledge and improve the quality of care I provide, and I will render it with kindness, because I truly believe: there are no unimportant jobs, no unimportant people, and no unimportant acts of kindness.

The NAGNA mission is in fact, a fairly direct way nursing homes can meet OBRA Quality of Life requirements. How? Because as residents tell us daily their number one desire is to have a good nurses' aide, and a good relationship with her or him. NAGNA assures the high quality attitude of a professional nurses' aide will be present at the bedside, and thus OBRA compliance is that much easier.

ASSURING PROFESSIONAL PASTORAL CARE FOR EVERY NURSING HOME RESIDENT

In Vermont, we have 46 nursing homes, but only one facility has a part-time, paid chaplain. Owned by a hospital, the nursing home shares the chaplaincy position. Reviewing our history lesson, we know spirituality and care used to be inseparable, a package deal. For some reason, this concept was partially preserved in prisons, hospitals and even mental institutions, but it has yet to take hold in nursing homes. Today, with even more nursing home beds than hospital beds nationwide, the need for chaplains to serve older Americans is undeniable.

When I was a child, my father invented a rather crude but effective switch for our old black and white television, that we utilized whenever a commercial came on. My friends would laugh when Papa would yell, "hit the switch!" and we would snap off the offensive advertisement. "One day, enough people will complain about those blasted things, so the manufacturers will put a switch right on the TV," he predicted.

Well, enough people must have complained, because the mute button is now an entertainment staple. Is it possible to apply my father's formula to the need for chaplains in nursing homes?

Are there enough caring, concerned people who will call for attention to the spiritual needs of institutionalized elders? The baby boomers have driven most social change since World War II: women in the workplace, day care centers, even ATM machines. Maybe we can prevail on this critical issue as well. Chaplains who wish to take up the challenge can begin by approaching their local nursing home administration and politely inquiring about the following concerns.

- What were the results of the facility's latest survey?
- Are residents provided with hospice care?

- Would the administrator join the National Association of Geriatric Nursing Assistants?
- Would administration allow the chaplain to help the staff learn about the noble calling of caregivers, and possibly, with the financial support of a local church, host a workshop conducted by the Foundation for Compassionate Care?
- How is the death of a resident handled by the facility?

Chaplains can also approach the state survey department about requiring bereavement and death education for nursing home staff. Hopefully we can prevail on this critical issue and comfort all who mourn.

REFERENCES

American HealthCare Association. 1998. *National data on nursing facilities* (www.ahca.org).

Commonwealth Fund. 1996. *OBRA 1987 Report.*

Cummings, R. 1993. Foundation for Compassionate Care, 24 Colonial Dr., Montpelier, VT 05602.

HealthCare Financing Administration. 1995. Guidance to surveyors in long term care facilities. *Code of federal regulations*, section 483.15.

Hoffman, R. 1997. *Nursing assistant monthly.*

Johnson, C., Grant, L. 1985. *The nursing home in American society.* Baltimore: The Johns Hopkins University Press. p. 3.

National Association of Geriatric Nursing Assistants. 1996. *Code of Ethics and Federal Regulation Handbook.*

Nickles, V.B. 1991. Unpublished Masters Thesis. Appalachian State University, Boone, NC 28608.

Pardue, L. 1991. Models of ministry: The spiritual needs of the frail elderly living in long-term care facilities. *Journal of Religious Gerontology.* 8(1), 13-24.

Thompson, J., Goldin, G. 1975. *The hospital: A social and architectural history.* New Haven: Yale University Press.

Vermont Agency of Human Services. 1998. Developing community alternatives for the elderly and disabled. *Wise Investment . . . Improving Outcomes*, p. 36.

Vermont Ethics Network. 1997. *Journey's end: Vermont voices on care of the dying.* 22-27.

Vladeck, B. 1981. *Unloving care: The nursing home tragedy.* Ontario, California: Basic Books.

In Memory of Loved Ones Who Have Enriched Our Lives: Helping Staff Create and Hold Memorial Services in Nursing Homes

Sandra DeForge

SUMMARY. This article describes the introduction of periodic memorial services in a nursing home for residents who died. The planning process as well as objections and concerns are discussed. A sample service is described, including the letter of invitation to family members and friends of deceased residents. The article concludes with three sample "tributes" to those whose lives were celebrated in a memorial service. *[Article copies available for a fee from The Haworth Document Delivery Service: 1-800-342-9678. E-mail address: getinfo@haworthpressinc.com]*

Working as an activities director in a 152 bed facility for almost 25 years now, I have witnessed incredible changes in the kinds of patients who come to our home, their care needs, and the staff who provide the care. Over time, I have watched the number of mentally alert patients go from the majority to the minority. Furthermore, the acuity level of our facility's census has gotten much more severe; we care for individuals who 10 years ago would have stayed in the hospital until they died. Now, their days end here.

Sandra DeForge is Activities Director, Berlin Health and Rehabilitation Center, Berlin, VT.

[Haworth co-indexing entry note]: "In Memory of Loved Ones Who Have Enriched Our Lives: Helping Staff Create and Hold Memorial Services in Nursing Homes." DeForge, Sandra. Co-published simultaneously in *Journal of Health Care Chaplaincy* (The Haworth Pastoral Press, an imprint of The Haworth Press, Inc.) Vol. 8, No. 1/2, 1999, pp. 109-116; and: *Spiritual Care for Persons with Dementia: Fundamentals for Pastoral Practice* (ed: Larry VandeCreek) The Haworth Pastoral Press, an imprint of The Haworth Press, Inc., 1999, pp. 109-116. Single or multiple copies of this article are available for a fee from The Haworth Document Delivery Service [1-800-342-9678, 9:00 a.m. - 5:00 p.m. (EST). E-mail address: getinfo@haworthpressinc.com].

109

These changes have not been easy on our staff, particularly the frequency of death. Once a fairly uncommon visitor, death is now a familiar part of our routine. For the nurse's aide who has always prided herself on helping patients get stronger and have a good quality of life, this change is a tough adjustment. Busy caring for her other patients, the aide doesn't take time to grieve and deal with her own pain.

In 1991, while discussing this situation with our visiting chaplain, Rev. Bethany Knight of the Vermont Health Care Association, she suggested we make some time in the activities schedule to pause and give everyone a chance to feel the loss. She wondered if we couldn't create a Memorial Service.

When we first talked about the idea, I was skeptical, it seemed like too big and public a step. I like to think I have developed an ability to tune into the moods and attitudes of the many Vermonters who live and work in the convalescent center.

"Don't you think they will find it depressing?" I asked Rev. Knight. "I don't want to make them sad." "Why would a Memorial Service for residents who have died be depressing?" she asked. "Do you think you are giving them news? Do you think they don't know they are going to die?"

The more we considered the idea, the more my staff of activities aides, our volunteers and I began to think it was worth trying. After all, some months there were almost a dozen deaths, and such huge losses were hard on everyone.

Working with the nursing department, I began to plan the service, to be held on a Friday morning in the large activities room. Fridays, the facility always offers a worship service, often led by visiting clergy. Lucy Drew, a retired church organist, agreed to play some familiar hymns for the Memorial Service, and Rev. Knight offered to collect some readings and prayers.

It felt like I had the hardest job, that of collecting stories and recollections about the residents who had died, from staff, friends and families. The task wasn't simple. Not only is it always hard to get momentum behind a new activity, the subject of death wasn't an easy subject to discuss. Just talking about the Service with staff was awkward, and I was nervous, still uncomfortable with the words "dead and died."

Listening to staff and family members talk about a dear patient who had died, I took notes. I asked the daughters and sons and grandchildren and surviving spouses to tell me about what kind of stay their relative had experienced at Berlin Health and Rehabilitation Center. I also asked what the stay had meant to the family and to the caregivers, and combined all these notes with my own recollections.

Beyond collecting memories for sharing, we organized the decoration of the multipurpose room. Two large bulletin boards were covered with blue foil paper, with big silver stars sprinkled across them. In carefully cut out letters, the staff placed these words "In memory of loved ones who have enriched our lives day by day."

Invitations were sent out to all those who knew the 35 residents who had died in the past three months. [The body of the invitation appears in Appendix A.]

Pale blue and white ribbons were pinned on all guests as they walked into the Service. Many residents were also in attendance, and a handful of staff. We began with music and some opening words. Rev. Knight reminded everyone that while we had all grieved our losses privately, something important and special happens when people come together for such services."

"Imagine a huge pot at the front of the room. Today, we invite you to come forward and pour your cup of grief into this common pot, knowing that by sharing our grief we dilute the pain. We also ask you to pour in your cup of joy, for in sharing the treasured memories of your loved one, you expand your gladness, since a joy shared is a joy multiplied."

"In this loving community called Berlin Health and Rehabilitation Center, we grow close. Today, we gather: staff, residents, family members and volunteers, to pay tribute to those who have died. We are here because we have loved, and for that, we have been blessed."

She then read Ecclesiastes 3:18, and read off the name of our first loved one: "We remember Annette Hartley." I stood and read a short memory piece about Annette. Her daughter and primary nurse's aide came forward to light a candle and receive a ceramic angel. Quite spontaneously, they hugged. Instantly, we saw what a beautiful completion this event provided us all. A chance to say thank you and good bye.

We continued in this fashion, sprinkling in hymns and poems. Sometimes, a granddaughter or close friend would come forward and share a sweet memory. Sometimes a nurse or aide would tell a funny story. [I include three longer tributes written by activities aide Carol Griffith in Appendix B.]

Within an hour, it was over. We invited anyone to come forward and light a candle to commemorate any death they had experienced recently. Several staff who had lost friends, children or siblings approached the table and quietly lit candles.

One of the activities aides finished the service singing "One Day At A Time," and we all joined in. Afterwards, over coffee and goodies, laughter was heard and the sharing of recollections continued! To our surprise, our visitors were in no hurry to leave. The morning had been a happy one, a time of healing and closeness. Far from depressing.

SINCE 1993

Since our inaugural program in 1993, BHRC has hosted two or three services a year, as the nursing home becomes more and more a final home for seriously ill patients. We've had to adjust the format, because sometimes up to half of the patients who have died only lived with us for one or two weeks. While we make great efforts to care tenderly for this short term population, we simply don't and can't learn about them enough to reminisce. Instead, our chaplain reminds everyone of our facility's mission, and the staff then shares the responsibility of reading the name of the deceased, his or her date of birth and date of death.

We have compiled an eight page, ecumenical printed program of poems, stories and prayers, called Words of Comfort, that we distribute to all who attend, following the service. This program is periodically updated, as a family member or staffer writes or submits something we think has a broad appeal. Participants have thanked us for Words of Comfort, saying they shared them with loved ones who were unable to attend the service.

Each time we host a service, we get more comfortable, refine the ideas, add yet another reading or ritual. In fact, we've had to learn how to gracefully limit the length of memory pieces, as some folks really want to talk! Because family members often have to get time off from work to attend, we make sure the total program is no more than one hour. We've found that our staffers are becoming more and more at ease with attending the service, and saying a few words. Very few employees can get time off to attend funerals, so this in-house ceremony fills a great need.

APPENDIX A

Dear Family and Friends:
The Staff and Residents of Berlin Health & Rehab wish to invite you to a Spring Memorial Service. Our program is to be held on June 3 at 10:30 a m. in the Large Activity Room. This service is designed to honor the lives of residents who have passed away during the fall months. We believe it is important to make time for such a celebration, when we can come together and remember those precious moments spent with our loved ones, who are no longer with us.

Rev. Bethany Knight, of the Vermont Health Care Association, joins me in leading the service with my staff and volunteers, who will provide the music. We share memories, light candles and pay tribute to your loved ones. The residents have made ceramic angels which we will place on our memory tree as permanent reminders of lives well lived. Please join us for this service. Our chef, Buddy Longworth, will provide refreshments following the service in the living room.

If you would like to say a few words, we would be pleased to include you in this informal but personal service. You are welcome to bring any other relatives or friends who wish to come. Please call me between 9 and 4, Monday through Friday, for any further information. I look forward to hearing from you and welcoming you to the Spring Memorial Service.

APPENDIX B

GEORGE O'BRIAN

How can I or anyone else for that matter listen to Irish music without thinking of George O'Brian, especially when you hear "When Irish Eyes are Smiling," George definitely had smiling Irish eyes, well I should say he did once he got to know you. I have to say though it was "somewhat" of a challenge to get to know George but it was an enjoyable one.

Working in activities, it is part of your job to "try" to improve the residents' quality of life by getting them involved in things they might enjoy doing. So, I set out to do just that, but George O'Brian was not exactly what you would call a social butterfly. For the first two weeks he was here, I really didn't think he was even able to talk, he never did. I would stop by every morning to say hello and make small talk and "if" I was lucky all I would get was a nod.

One day I asked George if there wasn't *something* I could do for him and he said "yes!!" Wow I thought, am I ever making progress. I asked him what I could do for him and he very clearly said "Get out of my room and leave me alone!!" I was crushed, my first thought was fine! If that's the way you want it I'll *never* set foot in your room again! After giving it some thought I decided that George O'Brian was probably a very private person. This very well could have been due to the fact that he was a high ranking officer in the Air Force for 28 years, working for the Pentagon and also planning funerals for dignitaries. I probably wouldn't say much either. So then I decided to respect George's wishes and leave him alone.

I didn't want him to feel completely alone so after a week went by I decided to just stop in to say hello or good morning and then leave! When I did this George asked me where I had been and said he missed me. Now that was a real shock. He then asked me if I was Irish, if I was stubborn and did I have an Irish temper. I had to say yes to all three. From that day on, our relationship grew. I soon found out the way to George O'Brian's heart was via his stomach, especially with chocolate milk shakes, or corned beef and cabbage. Bringing him a tape player with Irish music sure helped getting on his good side. His very favorite song was "Peg O' My Heart." This, he played over and over and over! Then I found out the center of his life was his wife "Peg" and his children who he loved very much.

Even though it was for a short time, it was a privilege to have George O'Brian for my friend and I am very thankful for the time we did have. I was very fortunate that George considered me his friend also.

It was very rewarding for me to have George give me that big Irish smile, come out of his room to an activity or to just sit and have one of our talks. We came a long way from the day I got kicked out of his room. George is sadly missed but will never be forgotten, he will be remembered every time we hear Irish music.

NELLIE THOMAS

Nellie Thomas was a resident that you could *never* forget because she wouldn't let you. She made sure of this. Whenever I think of

Nellie, what I remember most is her wheeling up and down the halls in her wheelchair and saying "my name is Nellie Thomas," if she got no response she would say it louder until she did get a response and she usually did. I should say, she always did. This is why I'd like to use her name to tell you how I remember her.

"My Name Is Nellie Thomas"

N has to be for *Nellie* there definitely was only one, also for her "No, I don't want to do it."

E was for her endless *energy,* she had more than the entire staff.

L the "L's" are for the *love* she had for her family, for babies, and for those who cared for her, well, some of the time, and for her laughter, most of the time.

I is for her "*I* want to go with you," when she would see us leaving at the end of the shift, and again for her "I *don't* want to!"

E is for *everyone's* heart she touched and for *endurance,* which she had an over abundance of.

T is for the *twinkle* in her eyes and for the *times* she gave us, I won't elaborate on the times.

H is for her *heart* as big as gold and soft as cotton, *some* of the time.

O has to be for her *opening* and slamming doors in the wee hours of the morning.

M is for her *making* us stay on our toes and for *missing* her.

A is for *anyone* who dared to cross her.

S has to be for the *sleepless* nights and there were many, also for that big *smile* she would give us when she would go by us and *slap* us on our backside. Whenever the occasion arose and then she'd say, "I just *slapped* your _ _ _ (backside)" Even though that wasn't quite the word she used. Last but not least, "S" has to be for her incredible SPIRIT which there was *NO* limit.

This is what Nellie Thomas has left in my heart.

CLEM SCHLUETER

I'm sure I wouldn't surprise anyone here if I said Clem was my buddy, he was my special friend. But then Clem was everyone's friend, he was loved by all.

If I was going to tell you what made Clem so special I would have to tell you about his many fine qualities; he was kind, helpful, thoughtful, caring, loving, gentle, respectful and very polite. He had a sense of humor that always kept our spirits up. He was a gentleman in every sense of the word.

Clem was stricken with dementia, this was very sad and heart breaking for those who knew and loved him, especially his family, but even though Clem had dementia, he never lost any of his fine qualities. He was always thinking of others.

How can one think of Clem without thinking of Trudy, his loving and devoted wife? They were an extraordinary couple. Their very rare and loving sixty year marriage was truly an inspiration to all who knew them. It always made my day to see Clem's face light up when Trudy or his son Greg walked in. Clem's family was the center of his existence. He had so much love for them, his heart was overflowing. His most prized possessions while he was in the nursing home were two five by seven pictures of himself and Trudy. He loved the one where they were kissing. He always said it took years of practice to make it look good.

How can I possibly mention Clem and not mention trains or Milwaukee? I can't begin to count how many times we were to catch the train and go there. The last time was when he wanted me to go to a wedding with him. I asked him, who was getting married and he said he was marrying Trudy. I told him "Clem you and Trudy have been married for sixty years." He said he knew, but he loved her so much he wanted to marry her again. That was his loving quality.

One day, he told me he had just seen my father and mother and had a nice talk with them. I said "No Clem, I really don't think so, they both died some time ago." He then said, "I'm sorry, that's terrible for you, that makes you an orphan doesn't it?" Then he asked if I would let him be my special father because everyone needed one. And that he was, my "special" father. That was his *caring* quality.

SELECTED BOOKS OF INTEREST

At least three authors who contributed to this work have also written books directly relevant to pastoral care of persons with dementia. They are listed immediately below and the comments describe their content and viewpoint.

THE MORAL CHALLENGE OF ALZHEIMER DISEASE. Stephen Post. *Baltimore: The Johns Hopkins University Press, 1995, 142 pages.*

Post is concerned that individuals, families, and society may not possess the moral fortitude to deal appropriately with the challenge of dementia. As regards individuals and families, he asks, "How can affected individuals and their caregivers maintain 'the courage to be before the foreboding specter of dementia'? Seldom does human experience require more courage than in living with the diagnosis and the gradual decline of irreversible progressive dementia. . . . " (p. 1).

As regards society, he notes that "Among the several most urgent questions of our time is whether human beings have in place the moral and ethical signposts that can point toward a future in which those who are so forgetful will be treated with dignity. This book attempts to articulate these signposts" (p. 1).

[Haworth co-indexing entry note]: "Selected Books of Interest." VandeCreek, Larry. Co-published simultaneously in *Journal of Health Care Chaplaincy* (The Haworth Pastoral Press, an imprint of The Haworth Press, Inc.) Vol. 8, No. 1/2, 1999, pp. 117-120; and: *Spiritual Care for Persons with Dementia: Fundamentals for Pastoral Practice* (ed: Larry VandeCreek) The Haworth Pastoral Press, an imprint of The Haworth Press, Inc., 1999, pp. 117-120. Single or multiple copies of this article are available for a fee from The Haworth Document Delivery Service [1-800-342-9678, 9:00 a.m. - 5:00 p.m. (EST). E-mail address: getinfo@haworthpressinc.com].

The remainder of the book addresses both these personal and societal ethical issues that arise from our "hypercognitive culture," a phrase that other authors in the field have frequently quoted or adopted as their own. As in the contribution in this publication, Post argues that despite the hypercognitive viewpoint of our culture, persons are far more than memory and intellect. Only when we appreciate that fact can we meet the moral challenge of dementia.

FOR GOODNESS SAKE. Bethany Knight. *St. Joplin, MO: The National Association of Geriatric Nursing Assistants, 1996, 370 pages.*

What would it be like for you to be a nursing assistant in a facility which takes care of persons with dementia? It could be rewarding; probably it would be difficult. As this book suggests, it almost certainly would involve being overworked, underpaid, and underappreciated. Certainly some of your peers at work would be friendly, perhaps even friends. The residents with less progressed dementia could be warm, friendly, and thankful for your care; those with more progressed disease could be unpredictable and difficult. All require every bit of personal and professional skill you have available. And remember, you likely have very limited education, income, and likelihood of professional advancement.

What is it really like? Lori Porter who writes the "Foreword" to this book can tell us. She writes:

> No job is more noble or valuable than caring for our nation's elders, and yet far too few aides realize the greatness of their contribution. . . . I know, because I began working as a nursing assistant when I was eighteen and continued to do so for the next six years. I was constantly amazed that we nursing assistants were not considered to be humanitarians, worthy of the highest honors. I was amazed when comparing our level of commitment and service to the level of recognition we received, and I realized that something could and must be done to recognize you and me and all our peers who dedicate their lives to quality resident care giving.

And what would it be like if you were the supervisor of these nursing assistants? A major problem you would likely face is employee turnover—in some facilities it is 150 percent per year. Steady, dependable help is hard to find and even harder to keep.

And what could you do to support and encourage your supervisees? High on the list would be to buy each of them this book! Knight has written 365 one-page inspirational pieces for nursing assistants—one for each day of the year. It is, as the title page says, "A daily book of cheer for nurse's aides and others who care"; it provides encouragement and advise to those on the front line of nursing home care. Each daily reflection is devoted to a theme: (January 28: Tell someone about your commitment to work: May 6: Mind your business and bite your tongue: September 5: Accept what is.). Each piece seeks to be affirming of the individual, to build ego, to encourage mutual support among the aides. The guidance it offers is sound: avoid gossip, focus on helping, take care of the person rather than the disability.

If I were a manager of nursing assistants I would buy each of them a copy of the book for Christmas and insist that they read it regularly!

FORGET ME NOT. Deborah Everett. *Edmonton Alberta Canada: Inkwell Press, Ltd. 195 pages.*

Everett's book is grounded in her experience with her grandmother who suffered by progressive dementia (i.e., "hardening of the arteries" as it was called years ago) for 20 years. The book's content is informed by her educational process which focused on ministry to persons with cognitive and memory deterioration as well as her years of clinical experience as a professional chaplain in this clinical context. The major content area of the book is titled "Spiritual Care for the Afflicted" and includes theological reflection, attention to spiritual assessment of those with dementia, issues related to grief and loss, the role of reminiscence, and the place of the church. A second section gives attention to the spiritual care for the caregiver. As in her contribution in this work, Everett emphasizes the importance of giving pastoral attention to the family caregivers. A final section in the book explores ministry as responding to the reality of dementia. The book explores a wide range of concerns all the way from theological foundations for pastoral care to how she carries out her ministry. It adds to the contribution she and others make in this publication.

Larry VandeCreek, DMin, BCC

Index

See also refers to related topics or more detailed topic breakdowns.

My Journey into Alzheimer's Disease
(Davis), 51

NAGNA (National Association of
Geriatric Nursing Assistants),
105-106
(The) Nathaniel Wetherill facility. *See*
Long-term care
National Association of Geriatric
Nursing Assistants
(NAGNA), 105-106
Needs, accommodation of, 102
Nursing Home Community Coalition,
94-95
*(The) Nursing Home in American
Society* (Johnson & Grant),
90,94
Nursing homes. *See* Long-term care

Older persons
as prophets, 5
religious awareness of, 15
Omnibus Budget Reconciliation Act
(OBRA), 101-103

Pastoral care, Progressively Lowered
Stress Threshold (PLST)
model, 7-23
Pastoral interventions, 45-57. *See also*
Spirituality
clinical significance of, 45-48
diagnostic disclosure and, 49-50
prayer, 55
preventive, 48-49
quality of life and, 50-55
Patience, 40
Paul, Apostle, 35-36,37,38,78
Persisting assets, 62
Physical stressors, 21
Physician attitudes, 46-47,50
Playfulness, 26
Prayer, 16-17,51,55,69
as activity, 19-20
Preventive measures, spirituality as,

45-48
Productivity, as value, 33
Progressively Lowered Stress
Threshold (PLST) model,
7-23
assumptions and principles of,
12-13
dementia management in, 17-21.
See also Dementia
management
religion as part of, 13-17
Project on Death in America, 104
Pronouns, avoidance of, 17
Psalm 136,86
Psychophysical nature of human
beings, 31-34
Psychosomatic unity, 31-34

Quality of life, 50-55,101,103

Rationalism, 54
Rationality, as value, 33
Reagan, President Ronald, 59
Recharge Your Batteries program, 90
Regulatory issues, 95-97
Religion
aging and, 13-14
in dementia, 14-17
memory as aspect of, 29
Religiosity indicators, 55
Religious coping, 14-17,62,87
Religious diversity, 49, 66
Religious symbols, 66-68
"Remember" as word, 37
Reminiscence packets, 64,70-71
Respite, 4. *See also* Caregivers
Rest periods, 17
Restraints, 102
Rights, as concept, 35
Ritual, as memory aid, 66-67

Sacks, Oliver, 46
Self-determination and participation,
101-102

Spiritual care for persons
with dementia : fundamentals
for pastoral practice